The Elementary School Counselor's Guide to Supporting Students with Learning Disabilities

This unique book informs elementary school counselor practice in a positive way that changes the lives of students with learning disabilities by helping to engage them in their learning in an effective and concrete manner.

Through a comprehensive lens, this book gives elementary school counselors the tools they need to work with students with learning disabilities in a school setting, starting with an overview of learning disabilities as they apply to the role of the elementary school counselor. The second part of the book then explores these topics in depth with a step-by-step program for creating counselor-led groups for elementary school students with learning disabilities. The 6-to-8-week plan outlines how elementary school counselors can create and implement the program in their own schools, and is accompanied by worksheets and handouts to help engage students.

Exceptionally beneficial for elementary school counselors and graduate students in school counseling programs, it is a guidebook for counselors working with elementary school students with learning disabilities.

Mati Sicherer is a high school counselor who holds an EdD in special education with a focus on learning disabilities. She has worked in education for over 20 years.

The Elementary School Counselor's Guide to Supporting Students with Learning Disabilities

A Comprehensive Program

Mati Sicherer

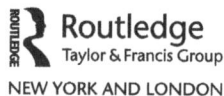

Routledge
Taylor & Francis Group

NEW YORK AND LONDON

First published 2021
by Routledge
52 Vanderbilt Avenue, New York, NY 10017

and by Routledge
2 Park Square, Milton Park, Abingdon, Oxon, OX14 4RN

*Routledge is an imprint of the Taylor & Francis Group, an informa
business*

© 2021 Taylor & Francis

Library of Congress Cataloging-in-Publication Data
Names: Sicherer, Mati, author.
Title: The elementary school counselor's guide to supporting
    students with learning disabilities : a comprehensive program /
    Mati Sicherer.
Other titles: Supporting students with learning disabilities
Description: New York, NY : Routledge, 2020. | Includes bibliographical references. |
Identifiers: LCCN 2020010734 (print) | LCCN 2020010735 (ebook) |
    ISBN 9780367430474 (hardback) | ISBN 9780367430467 (paperback) |
    ISBN 9781003000938 (ebook)
Subjects: MESH: Learning Disabilities--therapy | Child | School Mental
    Health Services | Counseling--methods | Program Development--methods
    Classification: LCC RJ496.L4 (print) | LCC RJ496.L4 (ebook) | NLM WS 110 |
    DDC 618.92/85889--dc23
LC record available at https://lccn.loc.gov/2020010734
LC ebook record available at https://lccn.loc.gov/2020010735

ISBN: 978-0-367-43047-4 (hbk)
ISBN: 978-0-367-43046-7 (pbk)
ISBN: 978-1-003-00093-8 (ebk)

Typeset in Baskerville
by Nova Techset Private Limited, Bengaluru & Chennai, India

Visit the eResources: routledge.com/9780367430367

This book is dedicated to all students with learning disabilities and to all of the people who care about them. As a counselor and a parent the task of trying to find that path for these special students was far more complicated and far less understood than I would have imagined. It is my hope that the work I did in researching and writing this book will help others to find that path seamlessly and peacefully.

Contents

List of figures

Acknowledgments

Of course, there are so many people without whom this book would never have been written. I have been so extraordinarily fortunate to have always been surrounded by remarkable people who have done nothing less than dedicate their lives to helping others. Thank you to my counseling colleagues (old and new) and all of the staff at Ryerson, Wayne Hills High School and Wayne Valley High School. Thank you to all of the teachers, administrators, supervisors, directors, staff, parents and students who make the Wayne School District the magical learning environment that it is.

Thank you to my sisters (you know who you are) for understanding that I needed to hide for a little while (again!) so I could write this book. Thank you to my whole extended family – all of you who I love and who love me back. And finally, my biggest and most noisy thank you to my family. Thank you to my husband, Scott, who inspires me, on a daily basis, to become a better person than I was the day before. Thank you to my three older children Andrew, Zach and Maya, who, as the impressive adults that they are now, encourage me to be as awe-inspiring as they are. Finally, thank you to Cass and Sydnee. From the minute these wonderful little humans entered our lives, they changed everything. They taught us so much about hope and acceptance and patience, and they took everything that I thought I knew about learning and replaced it with the questions that I hope I have answered in this book. Thank you all ... for everything.

1 Introduction

Why This Book?

In 2004, I was hired to work as a school counselor in a small kindergarten-to-fifth-grade elementary school in a suburb near New York City. The suburb was eclectic and bordered on one side by a narrow river. On one end, million-dollar homes sat on hilltops overlooking the New York City skyline. On the other end, closer to the river, bad drainage, lowlands and the swollen river after too much rain caused regular flooding in the trailer park and small houses that made up that side of town. The children who attended my school all came from the side of town near the river.

More than once did the people who lived near that river have to be evacuated, sometimes even by boat, and more than once did we have to send out flyers reminding parents that floodwaters were not safe to play in. The waters, which would have been contaminated by septic waste garbage, had the potential to cause serious illness, but since so many of my students' families were recent immigrants with minimal ability to read, speak or understand English, many times, the flyers went unheeded. My students came from places such as India, Syria, Turkey, Albania, Russia, China, Korea, Thailand, Mexico, El Salvador and spoke languages such as Arabic, Polish, Spanish, Albanian, Russian, Mandarin, Japanese, Circassian, Turkish and more. Others had roots in the United States that went as far back as the Mayflower. As the only counselor in the school, I was quickly thrown into the cultural mixed bag that was my school and I loved every minute. I loved the kids and I loved their families and I loved the staff and I thought that I was actually doing a pretty good job. I ran groups, I consulted with teachers, I met with parents, I ran workshops – I felt like I had a great handle on this very challenging and stimulating job and I loved every minute.

At the same time that I was beginning my journey in elementary school, my youngest children were beginning their own as well. Cass and Sydnee, my five-year-old twins, were just starting first grade. They had been in preschool since they were three and had attended kindergarten in the same building that they were to be attending first grade so they were already very familiar with school. They were bright and bubbly little girls who filled up with excitement about almost anything. They blazed with enthusiasm when we went to museums or zoos or even just to the park. For them, the world was filled with things to find and see and learn about. They asked so many questions about so many things that I found that I had no choice but to learn about them myself. After all, how could I could give them the knowledge about the world around them that they seemed to crave so much unless I knew the answers to the questions they were asking. And, oh boy, did they ever ask questions! "Mommy, why do the ants march in a straight line?" "Mommy, why does this bug curl up when I touch it?" "Mommy, why does the sun have to disappear at night?" "Mommy, why do we speak one language but other people speak a different one?" Their need for knowledge knew no bounds and I did my best to learn as much as I could to answer whatever answerable questions they had. They drank all of it in and remembered all of it. Strangers would often comment on my inquisitive and bright little girls and it would make me happy to see that their bright lights of knowledge were not just because I was looking at them through "mom colored glasses." At the same time though, I was also extremely concerned about them. Despite how bright I knew they both were, neither of them had shown any signs of the prereading skills that my other children had shown at this age. They did not recognize letters or numbers with consistency, and they grew easily frustrated when confronted with new learning demands. I had already approached both their preschool and kindergarten teachers and been told by all of them that they just needed some extra time. I argued with them all incessantly. How could they need extra time when they were so able to learn so much in so many other ways? How could they need extra time when I could see that there was something wrong? I was not convinced. I was an educator and a seasoned parent. My three older children had learned to read early and were already excelling academically. My babies, however, could not even spell their own names as they were entering kindergarten. Platitudes such as "everyone gets there at their own pace" or "it's not a race" made me crazy. I was well aware of the vast range that is considered normal for literacy skills, but I was also well aware of the fact that there was no reason why my daughters did not even have preliteracy skills at this point. They were inquisitive and bright and could synthesize verbal information better than many, much older children. We were also a family that read together all the time, which I knew was a great precursor to those early literacy skills.

Books were as much a part of our lives as breathing was. At the very least, my daughters should have been able to identify even just a few letters. They should have been able to point at an apple and say, even if they didn't understand what they were saying, "A is for apple." But they couldn't. They not only couldn't identify letters but they had also started running away from anything that had to do with learning to read or count. They were starting to become "discipline problems" at story time. They would cause a commotion or refuse to come sit with the group and I knew, despite the "experts" around me telling me not to worry, that there was, indeed, something to worry about.

By the middle of my daughters' first-grade year, I had expressed enough concern to finally have them evaluated by the child study team. At first, the team was resistant to doing an evaluation. At that time, the school district where we lived was using a discrepancy model as their primary tool for classification. This meant that there had to be a "significant" discrepancy between their ability and their output. A student, in the early grades, would have to have a significant deficit in order to be eligible for special education, and they suggested that we table the evaluation for a year. If my daughters did have a learning disability, they said, the discrepancy would get wider in second grade and this would show in the testing, whereas if we did it now, there would most likely not be enough of a discrepancy to allow for services. I nodded vigorously and agreed with the study team. Yes, another year would widen the gap. They were right about that. But who would want that? A wider gap might mean that my daughters would be eligible for special education but to what end? How much farther behind would they be after another year? How much harder would it be to help them catch up then? I pointed out research that indicated that the earlier children are identified and served through special education, the more likely it is that they would be able to read at a normal grade level later down the road (Abreu-Ellis, Ellis, & Hayes, 2009). I also pointed out that based on a response-to-intervention model (which was supposed to have been the primary model for eligibility, even at that time), it would have clearly earmarked them for services since they had not had any significant academic growth since kindergarten. I must have argued my case well enough because the team decided to go ahead with the testing. Even without a response-to-intervention model, the testing proved that my daughters were clearly eligible for special education services. It may have been a surprise to the team but it was no surprise to me when the evaluation revealed that my daughters had significant reading, writing and mathematics deficits. My daughters were classified under the "specific learning disability" category and were placed into an out-of-class replacement program (which our district called "resource room") for much of their day. They were there for math and for reading, but they returned to their general education placement for everything else. What this meant in practice was that for reading and math time, teachers were able to teach my daughters at the pace they required in order to fill in those missing pieces. For everything else however, they were back in the general education classroom where, even with modifications and accommodations, they were still taught at the same pace and in the same manner as their peers.

This mix of special and general education was supposed to make my daughters feel included while still giving them the education they required in order to learn. Yes, my daughters got taught at a different pace and with different modalities in the resource room, and yes, they had multiple modifications and accommodations for all of their general education subject areas, but something was still very wrong. Before they were classified, they were angry and frustrated because they wanted so much to learn just like all the other children and could not seem to do it. They would sit in class and try to hide how much they did not know and wonder why it was that they were so different from their peers. Once they started receiving special education services, I thought everything would get better, but I was so very wrong. That anger and frustration did not go away. In fact, it seemed to increase in intensity. Although they were very, very slowly starting to make some progress, they hated being taken out of their general education classroom each day during reading and math time. To them, this daily intrusion into their classroom was a blatant sign that they were struggling. Whereas before, they were upset because they were struggling, now they were upset because they were struggling but everyone else knew it too. Everyone knew that the students who were being pulled out of the class for this extra help were "special" so suddenly their deficits had become much more public. The daily routine of leaving their classroom for the resource room was an exercise in humiliation for them. Being pulled out of their general education class and into the "special" class may have helped them start to learn but it also seemed to solidify their differences in a very negative way. They were not like most of their peers. To make matters worse, their resource room serviced students with all ranges of cognitive challenges. They would look at their classmates in their general education class and then at their classmates in their resource room class and ask me constantly why, if they were as smart as I kept telling them they were, they kept getting pulled out of the class where the "smart" kids were. Why, they wondered, if they were so smart, could they not learn just like the other "smart" children?

To make matters even more difficult, when they did stay in their general education class for subjects other than math or reading, they could still not follow along. Each day that passed when a teacher told them to open their social studies book and read a passage or gave them a homework assignment based on work that they had already not understood during their school day was another reason to think that they were something less than their peers and all of this seemed to solidify the negative self-concept that they already had about their ability to learn.

They continued to progress slowly in the resource room but they also continued to feel terrible about themselves as learners and feel disenfranchised as members of their class. They didn't feel like they belonged anywhere and no one addressed any of it. No one talked about their learning disabilities. It was as if once they were placed in the resource room, all conversation about what got them there and what it meant, or what it might mean later on, just suddenly stopped. Aside from two gifted and beautiful teachers who were able to see each and every child as the gift that they were (thank you Mrs. Recca and Mrs. Clark!), no one addressed my daughters' challenges in the context of their strengths and I was starting to see some worrisome signs. I found a tuft of hair on the bathroom counter and realized that one of them had been pulling out her hair. They were both biting their nails so far down that their fingers just looked like bloody little stumps. Most worrisome was that fact that they just seemed to be losing interest in the things they used to love.

Sydnee had always loved learning about science and Cass had always loved to draw, but neither one of them seemed to want any of that any longer. They cried a lot. At homework time, they banged their heads against the wall and called themselves stupid. They did not seek out friends, nor were they sought out by other children. I knew they were getting the academic support they needed, but something still continued to be very, very wrong. They hated reading. They hated homework. They hated the resource room and they hated the general education classroom.

Even though they were starting to read, they knew they were still far behind their peers and to them this still translated as failure. How could they be getting what they needed but still be feeling so terrible? I started having nightmares every night. I dreamt about them growing up angry and unable to read or add or subtract. I was growing more and more scared every day. I could see that my beautiful, brilliant and happy little girls might be heading down a path of educational disengagement and depression, and there was just no world in which I would allow these two special little girls to become anything other than the students that they had always wanted to be, but I was stuck and did not know what I could do to help them. The day I heard sobs coming from their room and saw my youngest daughter on the floor surrounded by books she could not read and screaming that she would never be anything but stupid was the turning point for me.

I knew that how students feel about school and themselves as students has an effect on how well they perform (Lane, Lane, & Kyprianou, 2004). I also knew that there was no way I was going to let these two little girls who had, up to now, wanted to know everything about everything, lose their self-esteem, motivation or interest in learning. It didn't matter if no one in my daughters' educational life knew how to help them. It didn't even matter if I didn't know how to help them because I was going to learn. Since I was already an educator with a master's degree in counseling, I was already ahead of the game. I took a deep breath and dove in.

I started by doing extensive research about their learning disabilities. I taught myself everything I could learn about dyslexia and then I taught them whatever I had learned. We read stories about famous and successful people with learning disabilities. We discussed how learning disabilities did not define intelligence. We even discussed how most people had no understanding of what dyslexia actually was and how important it was for them to educate people about it when they saw that people around them misunderstood their disability. It was a good start but it was not enough.

By the end of third grade, my daughters had finally learned how to read. They had not only learned how to read but they had actually surpassed their third-grade reading level. But it was not enough. As I found out, their difficulty with reading was only a part of their disability. Learning to read took care of learning to read but did not address their math skills, their writing skills, their visual or auditory processing skills, their attention, their social skills or their self-esteem. They were happy to have learned to read but there was so much more to cover, and in the end, learning to read seemed to feel more like a consolation prize than the gold medal we had all expected it might feel like. They felt different from their peers, they felt less capable, less intelligent and less bonded to their classmates. They were convinced that their classmates viewed them as stupid and I wasn't sure that they were wrong.

I knew how smart and capable they were. I could see the effortless way they understood verbal concepts that even my older children had difficulty with. If, however, you took those concepts and put them on paper and sat them down and asked them to solve the problem, or write a paragraph about it, they would shut down explosively and completely. As an example, one day, my middle daughter was struggling mightily with the concept of fractions. We were sitting at the dining room table and I was breaking cookies in half and in quarters to show her what the concept of ½ and ¼ looked like. Sydnee walked past us on her on the way to the kitchen, took one of the quartered cookies, broke it in half again and said, "Oh, I see! And one half of a quarter is one eighth of it!" Had the homework been hers, had she been sitting at the table trying to figure out the answer, I am certain that she would not have been able to do it.

This incident led me to start to question everything about their educational program including their general education placement and the homework that they were assigned. More research, more reading and more experimenting with what did and did not work helped to formulate a plan. My goal for my daughters was, of course, to make sure that they learned how to read and write and calculate numbers, but more important, it was to keep them engaged in learning and in school in a positive way. I saw that there was a point that I needed to push in order for them to keep moving forward with their learning. Each day was a tightrope walk between keeping their spirits up, keeping frustration at bay and pushing them enough to keep learning and feeling good about themselves. It was exhausting and necessary and terrifying, but if I didn't do it, no one would. The plan formed around the following ideas:

1.   Students who have an advocate who believes in them fiercely, understands their needs and fights for them tend to have more successful outcomes than students who don't (Muter & Snowling, 2009).
2.   For my girls, since I would be that person, home needed to be a safe place where their confidence was nurtured and their strengths were valued above their challenges (Wadlington & Wadlington, 2005).

3. Classwork and homework were counterproductive if there was no inherent opportunity for success in doing it (Cooper & Valentine, 2001).
4. Classwork and homework need to be evaluated for what they are actually assessing and modified appropriately both at home and at school (Cooper & Valentine, 2001).
5. Pushing them past their comfort zone was going to be necessary in order for them to keep growing academically (Applebaum, 2017). Being uncomfortable (without shutting down) was a necessary part of learning something new and a skill they needed to master (Applebaum, 2017).

I started with homework. Each night, as we reviewed their homework, I asked myself questions such as, Was this homework supposed to solidify the day's learning? If so, and if they didn't learn the information during the day, is this hurting or helping? Is there anything in this work that will make them feel successful or is all of this simply too much for them right now? If they were being asked to display mastery of a subject, was the way in which they were being asked to do it hurting or helping? If it was hurting, what was an alternate format that we could use to have them display mastery? If they could not feel competent with their own written answers, they would dictate and I would scribe their responses for them. If a worksheet was visually overstimulating and they could not focus on the problems, I would redo the worksheet for them to make it cleaner and easier for them to process. If they were asked to read a passage and they could not do it on their own yet, we would do it together. If there was something they simply could not do, I would ask the teacher to back off on this type of homework until they were more able to do it.

For classwork, implementing my plan was a little more difficult. Despite their individualized education plans (IEPs) and the modifications and accommodations that they were getting, their academic plan seemed based more on rote, prewritten plans than on my children's actual academic needs. When I asked for teachers to allow them alternate methods of displaying mastery or asked them to help my daughters access the learning in ways that were appropriate given their disabilities, I was told that they already were. I requested so many changes to their IEPs during this period that I know that their case manager knew my phone number by heart. I also learned, during this process, that the people who I was supposed to trust with leading my daughters through their education were not always as knowledgeable about their disabilities as I would have expected them to be.

Teachers did not always understand the depth and nuances of the learning disabilities my daughters had. They did not understand how I could simultaneously ask for them to lay off the homework for a bit while also asking them to accept nothing less than the best my daughters could do. I am certain they thought I was completely out of my mind, but I did not care. I am also certain that they just had no idea how to handle the multifaceted issues of learning disabilities.

One particular instance stands clearly in my memory. Sydnee was in fourth grade and in addition to her diagnosis of dyslexia, she had also just recently been diagnosed with inattentive attention deficit hyperactivity disorder (ADHD) and had also been identified as what they called "twice exceptional," which meant that she was both gifted and learning disabled. In her resource room class, she struggled with understanding numbers and was still catching up with learning to read, but she was also just starting to feel good about her intelligence and being in school. In her general education classroom, where, with modifications, she was expected to participate in classes such as history and science, she seemed to catch on to and synthesize ideas before the teacher even finished talking. This translated into her being in this no man's land of her being able to understand the bigger picture more quickly than her peers yet not being able to attend to the details, such as reading the textbook. She could explain something like why certain chemicals might react with each other but, at the same time, could not add two-digit numbers or read at grade level. Neither Sydnee nor her general education teacher knew what to do with this. Sydnee's response, given her ADHD and her giftedness, was to lose interest and doodle or stare out the window until she was called on to answer a question.

In Syd's world, the concepts were easy enough for her to float in and out and still be able to get the answers correct if she were called on. The teacher's response was to call a report card conference with me to let me know that Syd was not paying attention in class. The conversation went something like this:

Teacher: I want you to know that I am giving Sydnee a failing grade for science and history for not paying attention.

Me: I don't understand. Is she failing science and history?

Teacher: No, not at all. She excels in these subjects.

Me: So, now I am even more confused. What exactly is she failing?

Teacher: Paying attention.

Me: She is failing "paying attention"?

Teacher: Yes. She just stares out the window or doodles while we learn.

Me: But if she is not paying attention, how is she excelling in these classes?

Teacher: She is staring out the window.

Me: But she is excelling in these classes?

Teacher: Yes.

The conversation continued in this manner until I took the report card with the F in "paying attention" and handed it back to her and said, "I'm not taking this home to my daughter. She is just starting to feel good about herself in school. She is just starting to feel capable. I know my child. This will demoralize her and could end her positive feelings towards school. She should not be punished for what she can't help right now, and making her feel bad about something she has no control of will shut her down again just as she is starting to feel good. I need her connected to learning and to school, and I need her to feel like this is a place where she is seen for who she is and valued for that. She is excelling in these areas. Let's leave it like that. When that grade is changed, let me know and I will come back to get it so that Syd can see how great you think she is doing."

I valued the input from this teacher and certainly, Syd's doodling and staring out the window were things that needed to be managed, but there was a bigger picture. I was not going to let my child lose her positive connection to school. I was not going to let her fall down that rabbit hole of failure. We would work on things in their time but there was no way that I was going to let anyone call anything that my hard-working, intelligent and capable child was doing a failure.

It was this incident that opened my eyes at work. I had not been doing as good a job as I had believed. All day long I was called into different classrooms for behavioral issues, social issues and emotional issues, and I was addressing them and responding to them reactively. I would talk to the student, calm them down, bring them back and tell the teacher that they were fine now. The next day the very same students would be back in my office. I began to realize that all I was doing was putting a small bandage on a gaping wound and I realized that I needed to start seeing things differently.

All day long, these students, whose teachers may not have completely understood how their possible learning issues might have translated into behavioral, social or emotional issues, struggled with being labeled as failures. Maybe they were struggling with reading or writing. Maybe they were having trouble paying attention. Maybe they were having trouble understanding numbers. Maybe their academic struggles became behavioral ones. Maybe, just like my daughter might have experienced, these students looked excitedly at their report cards only to find out that they were failing at something that they had no control over at all. Maybe though, for these students, there may be no one there to know enough about it to push the report card back into the hands of the teacher.

Even for myself, as a parent, I trusted the professionals around me to know more than I did. Even when my instincts told me that something was different about the way my daughters were learning, all of the professional educators in their lives said that I was wrong. It was only when I insisted that they be evaluated that my daughters got what they needed. Until then, to their teachers, they were just two little girls whose abilities were a little below average and whose mother believed that they were more than they were and that is how we were all treated. The evaluations, however, proved different. The extensive tests that were finally administered to my daughters by the members of the child study team revealed that both of my daughters had profound disabilities masked by high intelligence. It seemed on the day of their first IEP meeting, as we reviewed the results of the testing, that everyone in the room except for me was surprised to find out that my daughters were not two little girls with below average intelligence whose mother did not believe that they were more than they were.

Most parents do not understand learning disabilities. Most parents will trust the people who are teaching their children to tell them if there is something wrong. Most parents will take that failing grade on that report card and bring it home. And most parents don't realize until it is too late that they have chased their children into that rabbit hole of failure waving that report card in the air without ever meaning to.

The day I had that meeting with Sydnee's teacher and handed back that report card was the day I became certain that my children would be fine. I knew they would be fine because I would never accept anything less. I was willing to push report cards back at teachers, willing to be viewed as a pain in the ass by the child study team and willing to fight as much as I needed to in order open the doors of success for my little girls. But what about everyone else's little boys or girls? What if there is no one who can do that for them? What if those parents also don't understand learning disabilities? What if they are immigrants and don't speak the language? What if there is no parent at all? Who is the person who can work to make sure that every child, not just the ones who are lucky enough, gets their needs met? Who is responsible for those very same things I did to help my daughters? Those things were:

1. Advocating for children
2. Understand children's academic, social and emotional needs
3. Creating safe places where children's strengths are valued above their challenges
4. Working collaboratively with teachers, parents and child study team members
5. Teaching skills (such as the fact that being uncomfortable without shutting down is a necessary part of learning something new)

If this looks somewhat familiar it may because it is aligned with the 2012 American School Counselor Association National School Model (ASCA, 2012). We, as school counselors, are in the unique position of being trained to see and being able to have enough information to look at the whole picture of the child. Although we are mental health professionals, our practice is based in academic settings and as such, we cannot and do not separate the academics from the mental health component. We are, as school counselors, there to support the social, emotional and academic well-being of all of our students, and we are the people who need to step into this role. And this is why this book came to be.

Learning disabilities affect the whole child. They spill over the academic and land right on the social, emotional and behavioral life of the child as well. They are associated with depression, anxiety and negative behaviors. For us to be best prepared to support the needs of every one of our students, we need to be able to understand learning disabilities and how they manifest. If we are to be their advocates and their supporters, we need to be able to understand what we are advocating for. If no one else is there to have this understanding, and no one else is there to hand back that report card, it always, always needs to be us.

School counselors at all levels are in a unique position to be the agents of positive change in their schools (Dahir, Burnham, & Carolyn, 2009). The early influence of elementary school on student achievement places elementary school counselors in particular at the forefront for starting and supporting a positive academic, social and emotional trajectory. In fact, comprehensive elementary school counseling models have been shown to have a direct impact on higher achievement test scores (Sink & Stroh, 2003). This relationship between an effective elementary school counseling program and student achievement creates an important responsibility for the elementary school counselor. If counselors can affect such positive academic change through a comprehensive program, then it stands to reason that this effective programming be available and appropriate for all children. Unfortunately, this is not typically the case. Current research suggests that a large percentage of school counselors are not working with students with special needs (Milsom, 2002), and those that are may not be trained appropriately enough to be able to help them (Geddes Hall, 2015). Given the fact that special education students comprised 13% of all public school students in 2015–2016 (Snyder & Dillow, 2012) and the largest group within special education (34%) are students who are classified with learning disabilities (Snyder & Dillow, 2012), this is an inordinate number of children who are not being served appropriately by their school counselors. These students are being consistently and systematically being left behind, and the effects of this are devastating.

On an academic level, students with learning disabilities have a much lower rate of high school graduation than do their peers without learning disabilities (Smith, Manuel, & Stokes, 2012). If they are lucky enough to graduate high school, we have seen that there has been a significant increase in college attendance for students with learning disabilities (Grigal, Hart, & Migliore, 2011) but, despite this increase, students with learning disabilities seem to graduate college at almost half the rate of students without learning disabilities (Cortiella & Horowitz, 2014). So it seems that if we can get them to graduate high school, then we can get them into college. We just have not been able to figure out how to keep them there. For children in poverty, whose rates of learning disability are higher than for children who do not live in poverty (Gartland &

Strosnider, 2011), their rates of college attendance and retention are even lower (Lacour & Tissington, 2011).

In terms of their social/emotional success, students with learning disabilities seem to have higher levels of frustration, depression, social issues, tic disorders, anxiety and self-esteem issues than do children without learning disabilities (Cortiella & Horowitz, 2014). These students suffer more bullying (Rose & Gage, 2017), get suspended twice as frequently as their nondisabled peers (U.S. Department of Education Office for Civil Rights, 2016) and are three times more likely than their nondisabled peers to drop out of school (U.S. Department of Education, 2011). As young adults, these students grow up to have lower future aspirations and less confidence in themselves than students without learning disabilities (Cortiella & Horowitz, 2014). One in every three young adults with a learning disability has been arrested (Cortiella & Horowitz, 2014). Within eight years after leaving high school, one in every two young adults with learning disabilities has some type of involvement with the legal system (Cortiella & Horowitz, 2014).

References

Abreu-Ellis, C., Ellis, J., & Hayes, R. (2009). College preparedness and time of learning disability identification. *Journal of Developmental Education*, 32(3), 28.

Applebaum, B. (2017). Comforting discomfort as complicity: White fragility and the pursuit of invulnerability. *Hypatia*, 32(4), 862–875. https://doi.org/10.1111/hypa.12352

ASCA. (2012). *ASCA National Model: A Framework for School Counseling Programs* (3rd ed.). American School Counselor Association.

Cooper, H., & Valentine, J. C. (2001). Using research to answer practical questions about homework. *Educational Psychologist*, 36(3), 143–153. https://doi.org/10.1207/S15326985EP3603_1

Cortiella, C., & Horowitz, S. H. (2014). *The State of Learning Disabilities: Facts, Trends and Emerging Issues*. New York: National Center for Learning Disabilities.

Dahir, C. A., Burnham, J. J., & Carolyn, S. (2009). Listen to the voices: School counselors and comprehensive school counseling programs. *Professional School Counseling*, 12(3), 182–192.

Gartland, D., & Strosnider, R. (2011). Comprehensive assessment and evaluation of students with learning disabilities: A paper prepared by the National Joint Committee on Learning Disabilities. *Learning Disability Quarterly*, 34(1), 3–16. https://doi.org/10.1177/073194871103400101

Geddes Hall, J. (2015). The school counselor and special education: Aligning training with practice. *The Professional Counselor*, 5(2), 217–224. https://doi.org/10.15241/jgh.5.2.217

Grigal, M., Hart, D., & Migliore, A. (2011). Comparing the transition planning, postsecondary education, and employment outcomes of students with intellectual and other disabilities. *Career Development for Exceptional Individuals*, 34(1), 4–17. https://doi.org/10.1177/0885728811399091

Lacour, M., & Tissington, L. D. (2011). The effects of poverty on academic achievement. *Educational Research and Reviews*, 6(7), 522–527.

Lane, J., Lane, A. M., & Kyprianou, A. (2004). Self-efficacy, self-esteem and their impact on academic performance. *Social Behavior and Personality: An International Journal*, 32(3), 247–256.

Milsom, A. S. (2002). Students with disabilities: School counselor involvement and preparation. *Professional School Counseling*, 5(5), 331.

Muter, V., & Snowling, M. J. (2009). Children at familial risk of dyslexia: Practical implications from an at-risk study. *Child and Adolescent Mental Health*, 14(1), 37–41. https://doi.org/10.1111/j.1475-3588.2007.00480.x

Rose, C. A., & Gage, N. A. (2017). Exploring the involvement of bullying among students with disabilities over time. *Exceptional Children*, 83(3), 298–314.

Sink, C. A., & Stroh, H. R. (2003). Raising achievement test scores of early elementary school students through comprehensive school counseling programs. *Professional School Counseling*, 6(5), 350–364.

Smith, T. S., Manuel, N., & Stokes, B. R. (2012). Comparisons of high school graduation rates of students with disabilities and their peers in twelve southern states. *Learning Disabilities: A Multidisciplinary Journal*, 18(2), 47–59.

Snyder, T. D., & Dillow, S. A. (2012). Digest of Education Statistics, 2011. NCES 2012-001. National Center for Education Statistics.

U.S. Department of Education. (2011). 30th annual report to Congress on the implementation of the Individuals with Disabilities Education Act, 2008. *U.S. Department of Education.*

U.S. Department of Education Office for Civil Rights. (2016). 2013–2014 Civil Rights Data Collection: A first look. Retrieved from https://www2.ed.gov/about/offices/list/ocr/docs/2013-14-first-look.pdf

Wadlington, E. M., & Wadlington, P. L. (2005). What educators really believe about dyslexia. *Reading Improvement*, 42(1), 16–33.

2 History

As school counselors, we are charged with the responsibility of supporting the emotional, social and academic health of all our students including students with disabilities. In fact, the 2016 revision of the American School Counselor Association position paper on students with special needs states the following about counseling students with disabilities:

> The school counselor takes an active role in student achievement and postsecondary planning by providing a comprehensive school counseling program for all students. As a part of this program, school counselors advocate for students with special needs, encourage family involvement in their child's education and collaborate with other educational professionals to promote academic achievement, social/ emotional wellness and college/career readiness for all.

It is obvious, based on this recent position paper, that school counselors are expected to work with every single student in their school, including students with disabilities. This position paper makes it very clear that we, as school counselors, are responsible for working with all children including children with disabilities. Viewed from the ethical and social justice lens within the profession of school counseling, the role of the school counselor with students with disabilities is an obvious one; we support all students in their emotional, social and academic lives, and work as leaders in our schools to bring about positive and lasting change (Holcomb-McCoy, 2007).

In addition, laws such as the Education for All Handicapped Children Act of 1975 (No Child Left Behind Act of 2001), later amended in 1997 to become the Individuals with Disabilities Education Act (IDEA) and again in 2001 with the passing of the No Child Left Behind Act, create a legal responsibility for all educators, including school counselors, to include students with special needs in the curriculum. For students with learning disabilities and related disorders and any child who is cognitively able to move on toward higher education, school counselors need to ensure that the same college and career counseling that is being provided to other students is also being provided to students with these disabilities as well, but again, this equity does not seem to be provided (Milsom, 2002).

The reason for this exclusion seems rooted in the history of both special education and school counseling. For centuries, children with special needs were excluded from obtaining an education (Rotatori, Obiakor, & Bakken, 2011). If they were lucky enough to be able to attend school with their peers, they faced humiliation and abject ridicule. John Carlos, the 1968 Summer Olympics bronze medal winner in the 200 meters and former professional football player, wrote in his memoir:

> I was the kid wearing the dunce cap in the corner at school. That's not just an expression. My teacher literally made me wear a dunce cap in the corner. Back then the word "dyslexia" wasn't even in the dictionary but dyslexia was my affliction and school was an exercise in humiliation. (Carlos & Zirin, 2011)

Those students with learning disabilities (who were actually allowed to be taught in public schools) were not being taught appropriately in their public school classrooms. In 1975, however, all of this changed withthe passing of the Education for All Handicapped Children Act.which created a baseline for equity in the classroom. The laws enacted were put into place in order to create an equal playing field for students with disabilities. After this point, students with disabilities, including learning disabilities, were included in public education. For students with learning disabilities, it was not until the late 1970s that researchers began to explore different teaching modalities to engender their success (Worthy et al., 2017).

At the same time, the school counseling profession was also in a state of change. The school counseling profession, which had begun in the latter part of the 1800s in response to the Industrial Revolution (Beesley, 2004), had been conceived of as a practical response to the vocational changes in the world at that time. The breakneck pace of industrialization created a brand-new need for specialized workers, and schools needed to keep up with those needs.

Students entering the workforce needed someone to guide them toward jobs and jobs needed to be filled. Hence the birth of the school counselor. For decades after that, the school counselor, although involved in character development at some level, was, for the most part, primarily involved in helping students with vocational planning (Paisley & Borders, 1995) and later with a focus on clinical services only (Gysbers & Henderson, 1997). Change came with the reauthorization of the No Child Left Behind Act (NCLB) of 2001. NCLB focused on providing opportunities to groups that had historically lived on the sidelines of education. Minority groups were to be given the same opportunities as other groups, and the NCLB was supposed to be the vehicle to achieve this. Of the five primary goals of the NCLB (which included curriculum and achievement goals), the fourth and fifth discussed school culture and climate, development and high school graduation, all of which were ripe to become the functions of the school counselor (Stone & Dahir, 2015).

So with all of these pieces in place, it seems that school counselors should be perfectly positioned to help these students succeed, but this is not the case (Haksiz & Demirok, 2016). As mentioned before, we are getting students with learning disabilities into college, but they are not staying there (Grigal, Hart, & Migliore, 2011). The reasons for this lack of success are numerous. Students with learning disabilities who are receiving substantial support through special education services may not be prepared for the academic rigors of college (Francis, Duke, Brigham, & Demetro, 2018).

These students may be in specialized classes with modified curricula or modified tests. The transition to college (where there is no modified classroom or modified testing) can be an academic shock for which they may not be prepared. These students may also not have been exposed to study or time management skills (Francis et al., 2018). Without these skills intact, any student, not just those with learning disabilities, will have a difficult time successfully completing college. Another potential downfall for these students is the nature of their learning disability within the lens of special education. Due to the confidential nature of special education, school personnel are not allowed to discuss, share or make obvious the fact that a student has a learning disability. Whether intentional or not, this lack of openness about a student's learning disability could be adding credence to feelings of shame that these students already have about their ability to learn. Young children, even as early as preschool, begin making the internal dialogue that marks the beginning of what could later become issues with self-esteem (Coplan, Findlay, & Nelson, 2004). For students with learning disabilities, whose self-esteem is already fragile (Carawan, Nalavany, & Jenkins, 2016), these mental scripts that they run for themselves can color their entire educational careers. For these students, a conscious decision to leave their learning disability behind when they go to college may be a reality. This action translates into these students' active decision to forgo the support that they may need to be successful in college. Every college has an office specifically dedicated to disability services and can offer services that range from extra time to assistive technology to specialized tutoring. For students who require these services in order to "level the playing field," the decision not to access the services places them at an automatic disadvantage, yet many students who have learning disabilities do not access these services in college (Newman et al., 2011). Many of these students may not even be aware of the fact that there is a disability services office on campus (Schechter, 2018). Finally, for other students who have learning disabilities, there is the fact that they may not even be aware of what their strengths and challenges are at all. Despite having an individualized education plan (IEP) or a 504 plan through elementary and high school, these students may not ever have been told what these documents mean, let alone what they mean in terms of their learning abilities (Anctil, Ishikawa, & Tao Scott, 2008). For these students, starting college without any kind of understanding about what their learning needs are creates a milieu where they may not only avoid support but would not even know what to ask for even if they wanted it.

So here we are, back to the elementary school counselor's role in all of this. The research is clear on what is keeping these students from achieving success. If we know that part of the reason these students are not learning study skills, then study skills need to be in their programs. If we know that their lack of time management skills is keeping them from being successful, then time management skills need to be in their programs. If we know that a lack of understanding of their disability coupled with the stigma and embarrassment of having a learning disability is getting in their way, then we need to help them feel empowered, educated and aware about what their strengths and challenges actually are, and all of this needs to be done early (Cortiella & Horowitz, 2014).

Unfortunately, regardless of what we know about what these children need to be successful, we also know, since these children are not finding success later on, that it is not being done. The historical transition of the profession of school counseling from the vocational counselor to the clinical counselor to the program-oriented focus of the modern school counselor, intersected by the changes in education law geared at educational parity, left the counseling profession in the dust from a preservice training perspective. School counseling programs do not include coursework on special needs (Geddes Hall, 2015) and they certainly do not include specific coursework on managing students with learning disabilities (Geddes Hall, 2015). In fact, research suggests that less than 40% of school counselor programs have course requirements related to special needs (Romano, Paradise, & Green, 2009). There are also no real suggestions from the research for infusing this type of coursework into the preservice training curriculum (Geddes Hall, 2015).

Despite our lack of training, we are still mandated by the law, and encouraged by the best practices of our profession, to institute inclusivity into our counseling programs, but even with the legal mandate, there is still an uncomfortably large percentage of school counselors who do not and the reasons for this are multifaceted. The lack of preservice preparation for working with students with special needs can create low levels of self-efficacy, anxiety, low morale and anxiety about working with this population (Romano et al., 2009).

For counselors who do practice inclusivity in their programs, the bottom line question is simply this: What is that you are doing that counts as inclusivity and is what you are doing enough? Perhaps you are making sure to give your classroom lesson at a time when none of the classified children are being pulled out for special services. Or perhaps you are making sure to speak to each child in the same manner, spreading equity and parity over the classroom like a counseling fairy godmother. Perhaps you make sure to read books that depict children of all colors and abilities. Or you might actually read the class stories that center exclusively on children with disabilities and perhaps this is how to address the issue of inclusivity. We are told that we need to be inclusive and you've done it. But is this enough? Is it enough to just make sure that students with disabilities are included in counseling lessons? Is it enough to read books or have discussions about inclusivity? The research does not seem to indicate that this is the case. If it were enough, if our lessons and interventions were actually enough, the staggering statistics of failure for students with learning disabilities might not be the reality that it is right now. Perhaps what we need to do is to start to understand the potential and positive impact that school counselors can have on these students. Perhaps we need to take this understanding and develop a more profound knowledge of how these disabilities actually manifest in the classroom and how they affect these children. Perhaps we can even go so far as to be able to consult knowledgeably with teachers and child study team members or even to be able to identify these children. Perhaps we can even develop programming directed at the needs that these children have that are blatantly identified in the current research. And perhaps, from there, we can move on to give these students the equity and parity that they actually require in order to become the successful adults that they have the right to be.

This book picks up where the changes to our profession dropped us. It gives us a framework for understanding learning disabilities and how they manifest in the elementary school classroom and gives us a roadmap to actually giving these students the skills that they will need to be successful.

References

Anctil, T. M., Ishikawa, M. E., & Tao Scott, A. (2008). Academic identity development through self-determination: Successful college students with learning disabilities. *Career Development for Exceptional Individuals*, 31(3), 164–174. https://doi.org/10.1177/0885728808315331

ASCA. (2016). The School Counselor and Students with Disabilities. Retrieved from https://www.schoolcounselor.org/asca/media/asca/PositionStatements/PS_Disabilities.pdf

Beesley, D. (2004). Teachers' perceptions of school counselor effectiveness: Collaborating for student success. *Education*, 125(2).

Carawan, L. W., Nalavany, B. A., & Jenkins, C. (2016). Emotional experience with dyslexia and self-esteem: The protective role of perceived family support in late adulthood. *Aging & Mental Health*, 20(3), 284–294. https://doi.org/10.1080/13607863.2015.1008984

Carlos, J., & Zirin, D. (2011). *The John Carlos Story: The Sports Moment That Changed the World*. Chicago, IL: Haymarket Books.

Coplan, R. J., Findlay, L. C., & Nelson, L. J. (2004). Characteristics of preschoolers with lower perceived competence. *Journal of Abnormal Child Psychology*, 32(4), 399–408. https://doi.org/10.1023/B:JACP.0000030293.81429.49

Cortiella, C., & Horowitz, S. H. (2014). *The State of Learning Disabilities: Facts, Trends and Emerging Issues*. New York: National Center for Learning Disabilities.

Francis, G. L., Duke, J., Brigham, F. J., & Demetro, K. (2018). Student perceptions of college-readiness, college services and supports, and family involvement in college: An exploratory study. *Journal of Autism and Developmental Disorders*, 48(10), 3573–3585. https://doi.org/10.1007/s10803-018-3622-x

Geddes Hall, J. (2015). The school counselor and special education: Aligning training with practice. *The Professional Counselor*, 5(2), 217–224. https://doi.org/10.15241/jgh.5.2.217

Grigal, M., Hart, D., & Migliore, A. (2011). Comparing the transition planning, postsecondary education, and employment outcomes of students with intellectual and other disabilities. *Career Development for Exceptional Individuals*, 34(1), 4–17. https://doi.org/10.1177/0885728811399091

Gysbers, N., & Henderson, P. (1997). *Comprehensive Guidance Programs That Work–II*. ERIC.

Haksiz, M., & Demirok, M. S. (2016). Evaluating school counselors' self-efficacy Perceptions regarding special education. *International Journal of Educational Sciences*, 15(1–2), 290–303. https://doi.org/10.1080/09751122.2016.11890538

Holcomb-McCoy, C. (2007). *School Counseling to Close the Achievement Gap: A Social Justice Framework for Success*. Thousand Oaks, CA: Corwin Press.

Milsom, A. S. (2002). Students with disabilities: School counselor involvement and preparation. *Professional School Counseling*, 5(5), 331.

Newman, L., Wagner, M., Knokey, A.-M., Marder, C., Nagle, K., Shaver, D., & Wei, X. (2011). The post-high school outcomes of young adults with disabilities up to 8 Years after high school: A report from the National Longitudinal Transition Study-2 (NLTS2). NCSER 2011–3005. *National Center for Special Education Research*.

No Child Left Behind Act, Pub. L. No. 1425, 107 (2001).

Paisley, P. O., & Borders, L. D. (1995). School counseling: An evolving specialty. *Journal of Counseling & Development*, 74(2), 150–153.

Romano, D. M., Paradise, L. V., & Green, E. J. (2009). School counselors' attitudes towards providing services to students receiving section 504 classroom accommodations: Implications for school counselor Educators. *Journal of School Counseling*, 7(37), n37.

Rotatori, A. F., Obiakor, F. E., & Bakken, J. P. (2011). *History of Special Education*. UK: Emerald Group Publishing.

Schechter, J. S. (2018). Supporting the needs of students with undiagnosed disabilities. *Phi Delta Kappan*, 100(3), 45–50.

Stone, C., & Dahir, C. A. (2015). *The Transformed School Counselor*. Boston, MA: Cengage.

Worthy, J., Villarreal, D., Godfrey, V., DeJulio, S., Stefanski, A., Leitze, A., & Cooper, J. (2017). A critical analysis of dyslexia legislation in three states. *Literacy Research: Theory, Method, and Practice*, 66(1), 406–421.

3 The Role of the Elementary Counselor

According to the American School Counselor Association's 2017 statement, the elementary school years are the time when students are beginning to develop their academic confidence, self-concept and feelings of competence (ASCA, 2017). Elementary school counselors use their programs to help support students' academic, career and social–emotional needs (ASCA, 2017). They also consult, collaborate and refer as needed (ASCA, 2017). This support has been shown to have positive outcomes in raising students' levels of academic success (Dusenbury & Weissberg, 2017). Given the fact that students with learning disabilities tend to have more significant academic, achievement, social–emotional, legal and employment issues (Cortiella & Horowitz, 2014) than students without learning disabilities, the need for elementary school counselors to begin a more laser-focused program for students with diagnosed (or even suspected) learning disabilities is great.

Current research points to the idea that intervention for learning disabilities done by age six has a greater likelihood of helping students achieve academic success throughout their lives (Cortiella & Horowitz, 2014), yet many students do not get properly diagnosed or receive proper intervention until much later in their academic careers. The role of the elementary counselor in terms of having an understanding of learning disabilities then becomes twofold: For the already diagnosed and classified student, the counselor can establish support and an arena for self-understanding. For the student who is struggling but may not be classified, the counselor can establish support but can also be an advocate for appropriate diagnosis and interventions.

Even though it may seem that elementary counselors have little to do with students' later college success, the truth is students' self-perception as learners begins as soon as they step into a school. The fact that we have been more successful at getting students with learning disabilities into college is overshadowed by the fact that these very same students are graduating college at almost half the rate of students without learning disabilities (Cortiella & Horowitz, 2014).

In order to help our students with learning disabilities become more aware and accepting of themselves as learners, counselors need to have a firm understanding of those learning disabilities. With this understanding in place, it becomes easier for us to help them begin to understand and accept themselves.

References

ASCA. (2017). The essential role of elementary school counselors. Retrieved from https://www.schoolcounselor.org/asca/media/asca/Careers-Roles/WhyElem.pdf

Cortiella, C., & Horowitz, S. H. (2014). *The State of Learning Disabilities: Facts, Trends and Emerging Issues.* New York: National Center for Learning Disabilities.

Dusenbury, L., & Weissberg, R. P. (2017). Social emotional learning in elementary school: Preparation for success. *The Education Digest*, 83(1), 36.

4   What Are Learning Disabilities?

As counselors, we are taught to understand and respect differences. We understand the importance of cultural and socioeconomic competencies, and we are trained to have empathy and inclusion at the core of our practice. Unfortunately, when it comes to students with learning disabilities, many of us do not have the knowledge base we need about these issues to be able to help out students effectively. Our lack of knowledge about these challenges leaves us at a disadvantage. It is difficult if not impossible to establish empathy, inclusion and understanding when we may not understand the basic challenges that students with learning disabilities face.

Our profession asks us to delve deeply into the why of things that happen. When we see a student who is behaving in a negative manner, we look for the reasons this behavior is happening and then we create interventions. When we see a student who always seems sad, we begin to explore the reasons behind this sad affect in order to start helping the student maneuver through their emotions in a positive way. The process of looking for the answers to these questions is the beginning of the process of getting our students the help that they need. As much of an understanding that we have about the social–emotional aspect of our students' lives is as much as we need to have about their learning disabilities. Learning disabilities affect every aspect of a student's life including their emotional and social states, their academic achievement and their career aspirations. As professionals in an educational setting, we need to be able to understand learning disabilities, recognize how they manifest and have a core knowledge of how to best guide these students through elementary school and beyond.

At the most straightforward level, learning disabilities can be defined as substantial struggles with reading, writing, spelling and/or math, despite average or above-average intelligence. These disorders are real. They have been recognized by the medical community for over a hundred years (Silver & Hagin, 1990), and when they are diagnosed, they are managed in public schools through a continuum model that can range from allowing extra time to complete tests and/ or assignments all the way to full-time placement in schools specially designed to address learning disabilities.

Reference

Silver, A. A., & Hagin, R. A. (1990). *Disorders of Learning in Childhood*. New York: John Wiley & Sons.

5 Most Common Learning Disabilities and Related Disorders

DYSLEXIA

In this part:

- What is dyslexia?
- What are some symptoms of dyslexia?
- What helps someone with dyslexia?

What Is Dyslexia?

Dyslexia is a language-based learning disability that is characterized by difficulties with reading, spelling, writing and processing at any level of intelligence and affects the ability to read (Tanaka et al., 2011). In an individualized education plan (IEP) it is frequently part of the "Specific learning disability" category.

A common myth about dyslexia is that it is a visual problem and that people with dyslexia see letters backward. Dyslexia is actually a neurologically based language processing disorder that, although it does not cause people to see letters backward, does cause difficulty processing and interpreting letters and words. Students with dyslexia have had difficulty learning to attach sounds to letters. For a student without dyslexia, learning that the letter "A" is attached to the first sound in the word "apple" happens almost organically. For students with dyslexia, that connection is at the center of a struggle to learn to read. Students with dyslexia have described looking at a reading passage as trying to decipher a foreign language. For these students, it is hard to reconcile their intelligence with their difficulty learning how to read.

Watching other students learn so seamlessly while they may continue to struggle with the basics can bring up feelings of frustration, lowered self-esteem, depression and anxiety (Cortiella & Horowitz, 2014). Without proper intervention, students with dyslexia can get stuck in a cycle of frustration that can lead to continued academic, social and emotional issues and, eventually, potential disengagement in school.

Although it seems unclear what the direct cause of dyslexia is, there are many things we do know for certain. When dyslexia is present, it frequently occurs in tandem with other neurological disorders such as dyscalculia, attention deficit disorder and dysgraphia (Wilson et al., 2015). Another thing we know is that it does not discriminate based on gender, socioeconomic status or intellectual ability (Macdonald, 2010). Interestingly as well, people with dyslexia can be extremely gifted in areas such as art, music and drama, although whether the reason for this is because of an intrinsic connection or as a reaction to having these academic difficulties, it is hard to tell (Chakravarty, 2009).

Approximately 15% to 20% of the population have symptoms of dyslexia, but not all of them will be identified for special education interventions. Many students with dyslexia do a good job of covering up their struggles and eventually just resign themselves to believing that they are just not smart or academically oriented. Other students, although they may have the disorder, are still not eligible for special education. Of the students with dyslexia who are classified, many of them are classified under the umbrella of "specific learning disability." These students with dyslexia comprise about 85% of all students who are classified under the category of "specific learning disability," and these students make up about 13% to 14% of all public school students who qualify for special education (International Dyslexia Organization, 2015).

What Are Some Symptoms of Dyslexia?

A student with dyslexia may:

- Have difficulty with linking letters with sounds, rhyming, recognizing simple words and hearing individual sounds
- Have issues with articulation
- Have difficulty counting syllables in words
- Have difficulty recognizing rhymes
- Look for ways to avoid reading such as sharpening pencils or asking to go to the bathroom
- Struggle with reading, writing, spelling, decoding and fluent word recognition
- Communicate better orally than in written form
- Be more tired than other students from the extra effort of attending and concentrating
- Have behavioral issues
- Struggle with reading charts and graphs
- Be convinced that they are "stupid" or just not "good at school"
- Have inconsistent learning; they will "know" something on one day but no longer "know" it the next

- Have poor concentration
- Struggle with learning and remembering new terminology
- Forget words
- Have difficulty understanding idioms
- Have difficulty following a sequence of instruction
- Hand in messy papers with many crossed-out words and the same word spelled different ways throughout the paper
- Have trouble completing homework
- Be confused by similar-looking letters (e.g., b and d)
- Reverse letters
- Have poor or unusual pencil grip
- Not produce work that seems appropriate to their ability
- Pronounce words in an unusual manner
- Miss or add words when reading out loud
- Have difficulty with supporting an argument or getting to the point
- Not recognize words that should be familiar
- Have low self-esteem
- Have difficulty remembering sequential orders (e.g., days of the week, months of the year)
- Have difficulty learning to tell time
- Be confused by directionality (e.g., right/left, east/west, up/down)
- Be withdrawn or the "class clown"
- Have difficulty remembering dates, phone numbers, birthdays, etc.
- Have challenges recalling names of people and/or places
- Struggle with learning a foreign language (British Dyslexia Association, 2017; Goswami, 2008; International Dyslexia Organization, 2015; Lyon, 1995; NICHD, 2017; Shaywitz, 2003)

(Note: Although many people experience many of these challenges, a student with dyslexia may exhibit several of these challenges simultaneously.)

What Helps Someone with Dyslexia?

- Having a class syllabus
- Access to recorded lessons
- Having teacher or student notes
- Monitoring of long-term assignments
- Audiobooks
- Access to a laptop
- Study guides
- Extra teacher attention
- Flash cards
- Minimizing distractions

- Breaking up big projects
- Access to outlines
- Access to diagrams
- Reading writing assignments aloud and then editing
- Speech-to-text programs
- Text-to-speech programs

DYSCALCULIA

In this part:

- What is dyscalculia?
- What are some symptoms of dyscalculia?
- What helps someone with dyscalculia?

What Is Dyscalculia?

Dyscalculia is a specific learning disability that affects the normal acquisition of arithmetic skills. It is, like dyslexia, a persistent and neurological disorder, but unlike dyslexia, teaching and environmental factors are also involved in its etiology (Shalev, 2001). It is viewed as difficulty with understanding and representing the number of objects in a set and more specifically with struggles in number processing, memorizing, reasoning and executing calculations (Butterworth, 2018). Dyscalculia has been shown to have similar prevalence as dyslexia (Chideridou–Mandari, Padeliadu, Karamatsouki, Sandravelis, & Karagiannidis, 2016) and seems to affect boys as frequently as it does girls (Shalev, 2001). It affects about 5% to 6% of school-aged children (Shalev, 2001) and, like dyslexia, has also been associated with prematurity and low birthweight (Shalev, 2001). Dyscalculia also frequently occurs in tandem with other neurological disorders such as dyslexia, attention deficit disorder and dysgraphia (Shalev, 2001).

What Are Some Symptoms of Dyscalculia?

A student with dyscalculia may:

- Have difficulty with word problems
- Be challenged when making change or handling money
- Show difficulty with concepts such as number lines, positive and negative value, place value, quantity, and carrying and borrowing
- Exhibit difficulty keeping numbers lined up for calculations such as long division problems
- Have difficulty with sequencing information or events
- Exhibit challenges when using multiple steps in math operations
- Show difficulty with fractions

- Display difficulty recognizing patterns
- Have difficulty understanding time-related concepts such as days, weeks, months, etc. (Shalev, 2001)

What Helps Someone with Dyscalculia?

- Extra time
- Frequent checks for understanding
- Clearly stated steps
- Allowing narration of math problems
- Providing sample problems
- White boards
- Connecting math to meaningful experiences
- Calculator
- Frequent review
- Finding patterns in the work
- Identifying and correcting errors after explanation
- Creating opportunities for success
- Frequent review

DYSGRAPHIA

In this part:

- What is dysgraphia?
- What are some symptoms of dysgraphia?
- What helps someone with dysgraphia?

What Is Dysgraphia?

Dysgraphia is a processing disorder that can be explained as an impairment of written expression. Although the disorder is primarily symptomized by the poor handwriting that seems to be its hallmark, its academic reaches go far beyond just that. The fact that it is a processing disorder means that dysgraphia is not just poor handwriting and can also manifest itself as difficulty putting thoughts on paper (Frith, 1985). There is also evidence that it can interfere with learning how to spell and write, and it has also been associated with dyslexia, attention deficit hyperactivity disorder (ADHD) and autism (Naser, Akram, Mandana, Afsoon, & Mehdi, 2016).

Students with dysgraphia may have very messy handwriting that presents with inconsistent spacing, unusual spatial planning, poor spelling and incorrect word choices. They may also have difficulty with choosing appropriate words and using grammar and syntax correctly in their writing. In addition, their writing may have word omissions or redundancies. Typically, these students perform at a much higher level verbally than in written form. For many teachers, receipt of that first written work can be something of a surprise, since the discrepancy between the student's verbal expression and their written work can be so vast.

Students with dysgraphia also often seem to display a tense posture and pencil grip while trying to write (Richards, 1999). This tense posture can exert these students to the point of what might look like unwarranted fatigue. In reality, these students really are exerting great energy in trying to process their thoughts into a written format, and this can and frequently does cause these students to tire very quickly. The fatigue that can be caused by this exertion then creates further challenges with learning to write and can create a cycle of failure that becomes difficult for these students to find their way out (Richards, 1999).

In addition to the physical act of writing, dysgraphia also refers to difficulty with aspects of written expression in general (Quillen & Gladstone, 2008). It has been suggested that dysgraphia is a dysfunction that creates difficulties with transposing mental language into written language (Naser et al., 2016). This means that aside from the mechanics of the writing itself, students with dysgraphia frequently may have difficulty with organizing their thoughts and expressing them in writing despite an ability to do so verbally. For these students, that act of thinking and writing simultaneously is a great challenge.

Current research about the prevalence of dysgraphia is mixed. Some of the current evidence suggests that dysgraphia affects about 5% to 20% of all students, but this number is not supported across the board. Other researchers suggest that although the prevalence may not be known, it is a disorder that is more than likely under identified (McCloskey & Rapp, 2017).

What Are Some Symptoms of Dysgraphia?

- Tight, awkward pencil grip, body or paper position
- Illegible printing and cursive
- Inconsistencies, for example, print and cursive used together; uppercase and lowercase interchangeable; irregular-sized, -shaped or -slanted letters
- Unfinished or omitted words or letters
- Inconsistent spacing
- Issues with previsualizing letter formation
- Slow copying or writing
- Unusual spatial planning on paper
- Complaints of hand pain
- Difficulty thinking and writing simultaneously
- Speaking words aloud while writing
- Avoidant behavior toward writing tasks
- Complaints about tiring while writing
- Poor organization of thoughts on paper
- Poor syntax and grammar

- Large gap between written ideas and understanding demonstrated through speech
- Spelling errors
- Very slow or very fast speed of writing
- Obvious frustration and stress associated with writing tasks
- Correlation with ADHD and autism (Mayes, Calhoun, & Crowell, 2000)

What Helps Someone with Dysgraphia?

- Teach compensatory skills (such as keyboarding) alongside remediation
- Specific and pointed instruction in forming letters
- Graphic organizers
- Occupational therapy
- Speech-to-text programs
- Teach proofreading
- Extra time
- Graph paper for math
- Early keyboarding instruction
- Remove neatness as grade
- Copy of notes

PROCESSING DISORDERS (VISUAL AND AUDITORY)

In this part:

- What is a visual or auditory processing disorder?
- What are some symptoms of a visual or auditory processing disorder?
- What helps someone with a visual or auditory processing disorder?

What Is a Visual or Auditory Processing Disorder?

Visual Processing Disorder

A visual processing disorder is a processing problem that can cause difficulty in making sense of information that is taken in visually. Visual processing disorders have nothing to do with eyesight problems. They are, rather, issues that relate more to how information that is taken in through the eyes is interpreted by the brain. This processing issue can affect perception and understanding of concepts, specifically in reading and math concepts (Brousseau-Lachaine, Gagnon, & Faubert, 2008).

Research on the etiology of visual processing disorder is mixed. Although there is no consensus across the board, there is some speculation that low birth weight and mild traumatic brain injury (Brousseau-Lachaine et al., 2008) are related to the development of visual processing disorder. On the topic of gender, it seems that the disorder does not seem to be affected by gender (Misra & Aikat, 2016; Molloy et al., 2013).

Auditory Processing Disorder

Auditory processing disorder is a processing problem that creates difficulty in making sense of information taken in through the ears. Auditory processing disorders have nothing to do with hearing problems. They are, rather, issues that relate more to how information taken in through the ears is interpreted by the brain. Since this processing disorder is based on a disconnect between what the student hears and how their brain interprets it, the act of sitting in a classroom and listening to a teacher is automatically impacted in a negative way. In addition, this processing issue affects speech and language as well. Since so much of learning relies on being able to listen in a classroom, process the information and create new knowledge, auditory processing disorder has a direct impact on the acquisition of all types of learning (Bamiou, Musiek, & Luxon, 2001).

Auditory processing disorder has a long history of research, and there is quite a bit we know about it. We know that approximately 2% to 7% of children have auditory processing disorder (Bamiou et al., 2001) and that boys are twice as likely as girls to have it (Roeser & Downs, 2004). We also know that auditory processing disorder may be related to prematurity, low birth weight, chronic ear infections and head trauma (Arky, 2018). In addition, there is also some speculation that children with auditory processing disorder are frequently misdiagnosed with ADHD due to what seems to be attentional issues inherent in both. The important difference between the two is found in the cause. Whereas ADHD is a disorder that is characterized by a lack of focus, auditory processing disorder is characterized by difficulty with processing what is being heard. This means that while a student with ADHD may not be paying attention to what is going on, a student with auditory processing disorder actually might be. The student with auditory processing disorder may look as if they are not paying attention but may actually just be processing the information too slowly or incorrectly instead. Even though auditory processing disorder has been researched intensively for many decades, it is important to know that some educators and professionals still express doubts about the diagnosis (Arky, 2018).

What Are Some Symptoms of Visual and Auditory Processing Disorders?

Symptoms of visual processing disorder:

- Difficulty with accurately perceiving objects in reference to other objects
- Difficulty perceiving words and numbers as separate units
- Difficulty with directionality
- Visual discrimination problems (color, form, shape, pattern, size and position)

- Difficulty reading charts and graphs
- Object recognition problems
- Difficulty with consistent recognition of numbers and letters
- Difficulty understanding whole/part relationships
- Difficulty with visual motor integration, and fine and gross motor skills
- Distractibility when presented with too much visual information
- Difficulty with copying from board
- Letter, number and word reversals
- Difficulty remembering phone numbers
- Frequent complaints of eyestrain
- May skip words or lines when reading
- Weak math skills due to omitted steps and confusion with formulas
- Difficulty with noticing obvious changes in environment (changed signs, displays, etc.) (Arky, 2018; National Center for Learning Disabilities, 2019)

Symptoms of auditory processing disorder:

- Difficulty in recognizing phonemes
- Difficulty with following verbal instructions
- Auditory sequencing issues (i.e., "tevelision" instead of "television")
- Difficulty with discriminating sound (words that are obviously different seem to sound alike)
- Inability to focus on important sounds in noisy settings
- Difficulty with reading and spelling
- Oral math issues
- Difficulty following conversations (especially in noisy settings)
- Poor musical ability
- Difficulty learning rhymes or songs
- Difficulty speaking clearly
- Social skills issues
- Comorbidity with dyslexia, ADHD and other related conditions (Johnson, 2018)

What Helps Someone with a Processing Disorder?

Auditory:

- Frequent repeated information
- Preview of information prior to learning in class
- Preferential seating
- Limited distractions
- Chunking of information
- Visual cues

- Clear and concrete directions
- Allowing for processing time
- Frequent checks for understanding
- Teaching note-taking skills

Visual:

- Chunking assignments into smaller steps
- Writing paper with darker lines
- Worksheets that are visually "clean"
- Allowing for alternative methods of checking for understanding
- Matching games
- Limiting copying from board

NONVERBAL LEARNING DISORDER

In this part:

- What is a nonverbal learning disorder?
- What are some symptoms of nonverbal learning disorder?
- What helps someone with nonverbal learning disorder?

What Is a Nonverbal Learning Disorder?

Nonverbal learning disorder is a language- and brain-based disorder that is characterized by challenges with nonverbal cues, spatial and visual organization difficulties, and poor motor skills. Many children with nonverbal learning disorder are frequently misdiagnosed with ADHD because the symptoms have overlapping qualities. These children tend to have precocious conversational skills, impressively large vocabularies and average to above-average intelligence, but because of the difficulty with nonverbal cues, they may have trouble making friends and maintaining age-appropriate relationships (Cornoldi, Mammarella, & Goldenring-Fine, 2016).

Nonverbal learning disabilities affect girls as frequently as they affect boys and also tend to run in families. The research is mixed in the prevalence of nonverbal learning disorder. Some numbers put it quite high (25% of students with learning disabilities), and others claim that it is extremely rare (Morris, 2002). Despite the fact that the disorder was first described in 1967 and much research has been done since that point, it has not been considered for classification in the *Diagnostic and Statistical Manual of Mental Disorders* (5th ed.; DSM-5) (Spreen, 2011) and seems to be inherently misunderstood and possibly underdiagnosed as well (Casey, 2016).

What Are Some Symptoms of Nonverbal Learning Disorder?

- Difficulty recognizing nonverbal cues
- Poor reading comprehension despite large vocabulary
- Very early and precocious language acquisition
- Gross and fine motor skills issues
- May appear clumsy and have difficulty using scissors etc.
- Frequent, repetitive questions
- Difficulty understanding idioms or spatial information
- Difficulty understanding sarcasm due to literal interpretations of events
- Difficulty handling change in life or routine
- May seem overly trusting due to inability to understand nonverbal cues
- May have trouble following multistep directions
- May have difficulty extracting generalizations from reading or real-life situations
- May have highly advanced verbal skills
- May have academic challenges in math computation, science, writing and reading comprehension (Franz, 2000)

What Helps Someone with Nonverbal Learning Disorder?

- Explicit and direct instruction
- Creating connections to new learning from previous learning or experiences
- Reduction of visually distracting information on worksheets
- Clear and concise verbal feedback
- Minimized distractions
- Frequent checks for understanding
- Compensatory skills instruction (such as keyboarding) and remediation (such as handwriting skills) simultaneously
- Occupational therapy
- Providing examples for problem-solving questions
- Teaching a variety of problem-solving skills
- Graphic organizers
- Speech-to-text programs
- Allowing narration of math problems
- Graph paper for math problems

ADHD (ATTENTION DEFICIT HYPERACTIVITY DISORDER)

In this part:

- What is ADHD?
- What are some symptoms of ADHD?
- What helps someone with ADHD?

What Is ADHD?

Attention deficit hyperactivity disorder (ADHD) is classified as a neurobehavioral disorder (Curatolo, D'Agati, & Moavero, 2010) that can interfere with a person's day to day activities and their ability to stay focused on a task. It affects 3% to 5% of American children and, although we do not know what causes it, there are certain risk factors that seem to play a part in its development. These risk factors include issues such as low birth weight, family history, cigarette use during pregnancy and brain injuries (National Institute of Neurological Disorders, 2018).

ADHD is characterized by at least a six-month period of inattention and/or hyperactivity and/or impulsivity symptoms that adversely affect daily life (Noorbala & Akhondzadeh, 2006). Although the disorder itself is not considered a learning disability, school-aged children who are diagnosed with the disorder may have difficulty attending and/or focusing on information that is being discussed in the classroom, and this difficulty in attending can have a significant and negative impact on learning. Early identification and treatment are pivotal in the prevention of associated later-life risks of social and behavioral issues, depression, anxiety disorder, substance abuse and associated learning disorders (Noorbala & Akhondzadeh, 2006). ADHD is usually diagnosed in childhood and is a lifelong disorder (National Institute of Neurological Disorders, 2018).

Although the disorder is officially known as ADHD, it is actually classified into three distinct subtypes. These subtypes are the hyperactive/impulsive subtype, the inattentive subtype and the combined subtype (Qureshi, Min, Jo, & Lee, 2016).

The student with hyperactivity and impulsivity may be viewed as having a disruptive presence in the classroom. They may be unable to sit for long periods of time and may appear restless. They may shout out answers or say inappropriate things to adults and peers alike without an awareness of consequences. Their loss of focus is frequently obvious and externalizes as hyperactivity and impulsivity (Noorbala & Akhondzadeh, 2006).

The student with a diagnosis of the inattentive subtype of ADHD, while still having difficulty with focus and attention, tends to display behaviors that are less externally obvious. These students may get distracted from a task quickly and easily. They may have difficulty finishing homework assignments or staying organized, they may lose things easily and they may have trouble attending to details (Noorbala & Akhondzadeh, 2006).

The student with a diagnosis of the combined subtype exhibits symptoms from each of the other subtypes in varying degrees (Noorbala & Akhondzadeh, 2006).

Although statistics show that ADHD is more common in boys than it is in girls, recent research has shown that girls tend to present with more inattentive qualities of ADHD and may frequently go undiagnosed. In addition, girls with ADHD also seem to present with more symptoms of anxiety and depression than do boys, and this can also lead to both continued underdiagnosis and misdiagnosis (Quinn & Madhoo, 2014).

ADHD is a highly treatable disorder, and treatment can help reduce symptoms. Treatments such as psychotherapy, medication (stimulant and nonstimulant), training and education about managing the disorder have all been shown to have a significant positive impact on adults and children who have the disorder (Noorbala & Akhondzadeh, 2006).

What Are Some Symptoms of ADHD?

Although it is normal to have some inattention and impulsivity, people with ADHD experience much more severe, frequent and disabling symptoms than people without ADHD. Symptoms for ADHD can appear as early as age three and may change over time.

General

- Difficulty with following instructions
- Inability to organize oneself
- Leaving projects unfinished
- Difficulty paying attention to details
- Poor academic performance
- Difficulty with relationships
- Social issues
- Disciplinary issues

Inattentive

- Missed details
- Difficulty with maintaining attention
- Easily sidetracked by other projects
- Incompleted projects
- Difficulty with sequencing
- Poor time management
- Messy classwork or homework
- Messy room, locker and backpack
- Difficulty meeting deadlines or being on time
- Avoidance of tasks that require sustained attention
- Losing unexpected things (coats in winter, glasses, etc.)
- Easily distracted
- Difficulty remembering to keep appointments
- Anxiety and/or depression

Hyperactivity

- Frequent squirming and fidgeting in seat at school
- Frequent leaving of seat unexpectedly
- Restlessness
- Difficulty with playing quietly
- Constant talking
- Shouting out answers
- Interrupting people while they talk
- Difficulty with taking turns
- Lack of inhibition
- Impulsive behavior (can become risk taking in later school)

What Helps Someone with ADHD?

- Consistent rules
- Daily routines
- Reduction of distractions for test taking, homework or classwork
- Direct instruction in organizational methods
- Direct monitoring of organization early on to establish routines
- Advance notice to prepare for transitions
- Extended time
- Shortened assignments at first to encourage engagement
- Color-coded notebooks
- Class notes
- Praise and positive reinforcement for positive behavior
- Acknowledgment of frustrations
- Nonverbal signals from teacher to help refocusing (Post-it note on desk, tapping on desk, etc.)
- Clearly written schedules
- Creating specific places to store frequently used items (keys in a box on the table, pens in a bin in kitchen, etc.)
- Homework and notebook organizers/planners
- Direct instruction in the use of calendars, lists and reminder notes
- Breaking down large tasks

DYSPRAXIA

In this part:

- What is dyspraxia?
- What are some symptoms of dyspraxia?
- What helps someone with dyspraxia?

What Is Dyspraxia?

Dyspraxia is a form of developmental coordination disorder (DCD) that can cause difficulty with fine and gross motor skills. It is a disruption in how messages from the brain are communicated to the body, and children with the disorder may have difficulty with coordination and motor skills (Portwood, 2013). Since the disorder occurs across a continuum, its effect varies from person to person and can change over time as the individual takes on different types of tasks and responsibilities. For example, when dyspraxia presents in a young child, that child may have difficulty learning how to tie shoelaces, ride a bike or even play with other children. As that same child grows into adulthood, those challenges may transform into issues such as learning how to drive or learning to make food, but ultimately, no matter how the symptoms present themselves, dyspraxia can impair day-to-day functioning. Problems with time management, memory, processing and organization are common and frequently result in difficulties with reading, reading comprehension and spelling. The disorder frequently occurs alongside other related issues and learning disabilities such as dyscalculia, dyslexia, and ADHD, and occurs across all levels of intellectual abilities. In addition, because the disorder can create such a negative impact on daily function and participation in daily life, people with dyspraxia also frequently experience social and emotional difficulties (Dyspraxia Foundation, 2018).

Dyspraxia seems to occur more frequently in boys than in girls, and there seems to be a hereditary connection, although no specific gene has been found yet (Lingam, Hunt, Golding, Jongmans, & Emond, 2009). While dyspraxia has not been associated with brain damage, it does seem to have a neurological basis and also seems to be related to risk factors including prematurity and low birth weight (Sugden, Kirby, & Dunford, 2008; Zwicker, Missiuna, Harris, & Boyd, 2010). In addition, recent research indicates that there is a 95% correlation between dyspraxia, ADHD, dyslexia and autism spectrum disorder (Richardson & Ross, 2000).

What Are Some Symptoms of Dyspraxia?

- Poor balance or clumsy movements
- Difficulty with motor planning
- Difficulty with coordinating both sides of body at the same time
- Hand–eye coordination issues
- Difficulty with organizing self and belongings
- Sensitivity to touch
- Handwriting issues
- Spelling and reading problems

- Distressed by loud or constant noises (e.g., pencil tapping, clock ticking)
- Difficulty with manipulating objects by hand (e.g., fine motor tasks, puzzles, cutting)
- Social and emotional difficulties
- Issues with time management
- Memory difficulties
- Processing issues
- Speech articulation difficulties
- Sensory issues from clothing (tight, rough, scratchy, etc.)
- Difficulty judging speed and/or distance
- Poor spatial awareness
- Poor stamina
- Difficulty adapting to new situations
- Literal use of language
- Difficulty remembering or following instructions
- Immature behavior
- Extreme emotions
- Lack of awareness of potential danger (Learning Disabilities Association, 2018)

What Helps Someone with Dyspraxia?

- Reassurance and acceptance
- Specific and honest praise on both effort and performance
- Reasonable and realistic goals based on student's abilities
- Early instruction in keyboarding
- Specific and constructive responses to work
- Extra time to compensate for slow processing of information
- Breaking new tasks and information into smaller chunks
- Allowing for time to practice
- Instruction of specific skills with an eye toward generalizing
- Step-by-step checklists for learning
- Verbalizing one direction at a time
- Minimized visual distractions
- Multiple modalities for teaching

EXECUTIVE FUNCTION DISORDER

In this part:

- What is executive function disorder?
- What are some symptoms of executive function disorder?
- What helps someone with executive function disorder?

What Is Executive Function Disorder?

Executive function disorder is a disorder that affects the ability to plan, organize, pay attention and develop strategies to cope with day-to-day life. People with this disorder show working memory deficits that affect the ability to plan and organize in advance. Children who have executive function disorder benefit from direct instruction and regular feedback about organization and planning. This early intervention is an invaluable aid to later life. In general, people with executive function disorder need help with managing time, space, materials and work. They need to be taught to use things like planners, timers and alarms. Although many people with ADHD have executive function disorder, they are separate disorders and can exist independently of each other (National Center for Learning Disabilities, 2005). A student with ADHD may have executive function disorder, but it is not necessarily always the case, nor is it always the case that a student with executive function disorder has ADHD (Willcutt, Doyle, Nigg, Faraone, & Pennington, 2005). If the executive function disorder is related to the ADHD, medication therapy might have a real and positive impact. If, however, the executive function disorder is related to a learning disability, medication therapy may not help, since in that case, the issue revolves less around loss of focus and more around a direct learning disability.

Executive function disorder tends to run in families and affects girls as much as it affects boys (Skogli, Teicher, Andersen, Hovik, & Øie, 2013). Since the disorder is characterized by difficulties with planning and organizing, the disorder does not become obvious until children enter school and the demands of projects, homework and schoolwork begin to be more prevalent.

What Are Some Symptoms of Executive Function Disorder?

- Difficulty making plans
- Difficulty keeping track of time
- Difficulty keeping track of more than one thing at a time
- Inability to finish work on time
- Difficulty planning long-range projects
- Difficulty communicating details sequentially
- Difficulty with memorizing and retrieval
- Difficulty starting tasks (Semrud-Clikeman, Pliszka, & Liotti, 2008)

What Helps Someone with Executive Function Disorder?

- Step-by-step instructions
- Routines
- Prior access to contents of lesson
- Frequent checks for understanding
- Clear and concise directions, given one step at a time

- To-do lists/checklists
- Chunking information into smaller bits
- Speech-to-text software
- Breaking large goals into smaller parts
- Timers for planned breaks
- Planners
- Direct instruction in the use of organizational materials
- Rewards
- Mnemonic devices

MEMORY ISSUES

In this part:

- Overview
- Working memory
  - What are working memory issues?
  - What are some symptoms of working memory issues?
  - What helps someone with working memory issues?
- Short-term memory
  - What are short-term memory issues?
  - What are some symptoms of short-term memory issues?
  - What helps someone with short-term memory issues?

Overview

Memory is composed of multiple moving parts, and these different kinds of memory are interconnected. The dependence these interconnected parts have on each other is an important component of learning. A breakdown in one aspect can have serious effects on any or all of the others. The ability to keep information readily accessible for new learning (working memory) can affect the ability to integrate new tasks later on (Learning Disabilities Association, 2018). Therefore, memory issues, although not directly viewed as learning disorders, can have serious and detrimental effects on learning at all levels.

Working Memory

What Are Working Memory Issues?

Working memory is the part of memory that holds information briefly in order to learn new things. It is the ability to hold onto little chunks of information until that information is able to turn into a complete concept. The briefly stored memory may eventually become part of long-term memory, but the brief hold of it allows us to engage in daily activities, such as following directions or driving, successfully. Students and adults with working memory issues have a difficult time following a sequence of directions and following through on tasks (Cowan, 2008; Holmes, Gathercole, & Dunning, 2010; Rosen, 2018). The working memory deficit makes it difficult if not impossible to hold onto the separate little chunks of information that later become the whole of learning. For example, a student with a working memory deficit who is learning the alphabet may have difficulty remembering the individual sounds that the letters represent and may therefore have a delay in learning how to read later on.

Working memory issues affect approximately 15% of children. More than 80% of these children struggle to learn in both reading and mathematics. There is some evidence to suggest that this group of children has academic difficulties that do not typically get identified for special education intervention. These children may have issues with sustaining attention, solving problems, and planning for long- or short-range projects or goals. These students may benefit from direct interventions in the classroom and direct working memory interventions (Holmes et al., 2010).

What Are Some Symptoms of Working Memory Issues?

- Quiet affect in large groups
- Inattention and distraction
- Issues with executive function
- Difficulty with planning
- Problem-solving difficulties
- Issues with sustaining attention
- Trouble with following through on directions even if the directions are understood
- Difficulty with multiple-step math calculations
- Word problem difficulties
- Reading comprehension issues
- Writing composition difficulties
- Difficulty with higher-order thinking tasks (Holmes et al., 2010; Kail & Hall, 2001)

What Helps Someone with Working Memory Issues?

- Compensatory strategy instruction
- Written sequential steps for problem-solving
- Written schedules
- Connecting new ideas to older and more familiar ones
- Chunking information into smaller segments
- Extra time for review

- Extra academic support for new learning tasks
- Modeling steps
- Checking for understanding

Short-Term Memory

What Are Short-Term Memory Issues?

Short-term memory issues are problems with retention of information that is only needed for a short period of time (Learning Disabilities Association, 2018). This kind of information, such as the recollection of a verbal telephone number, can be held for a short time or can be repeated and committed to memory to be accessed through long-term memory. Short-term memory is different from working memory in that it is just one component of working memory (Baddeley, 1966). Working memory is more about the entire process of taking pieces of information and converting them into learning. Short-term memory, however, refers to the process of short-term storage of information. This information could be temporary or could become incorporated into long-term memory as well. Students with short-term memory issues will have difficulty learning new concepts if there is a deficit in short-term memory (Gathercole, Hitch, & Martin, 1997).

What Are Some Symptoms of Short-Term Memory Issues?

- Difficulties in speech and language
- Difficulties with multistep math problems
- Difficulty remembering what was just heard (Alexander, 2004)

What Helps Someone with Short-Term Memory Issues?

- Lists/checklists
- Calendars
- Mnemonic devices
- Open-note or open-book exams
- Multisensory teaching approach
- Use of computers
- Routines and habits
- Repetition

References

Alexander, T. (2004). Memory/Recall Difficulties. Retrieved from Strategies for Creating Inclusive Programmes of Study website: https://scips.worc.ac.uk/challenges/memory/

Arky, B. (2018). Understanding Visual Processing Issues. Retrieved from https://www. understood.org/en/learning-attention-issues/child-learning-disabilities/ visual-processing-issues/understanding-visual-processing-issues

Baddeley, A. D. (1966). Short-term memory for word sequences as a function of acoustic, semantic and formal similarity. *Quarterly Journal of Experimental Psychology*, 18(4), 362–365. https://doi.org/10.1080/14640746608400055

Bamiou, D., Musiek, F., & Luxon, L. (2001). Aetiology and clinical presentations of auditory processing disorders—A review. *Archives of Disease in Childhood*, 85, 361–365. https://doi.org/10.1136/adc.85.5.361

British Dyslexia Association. (2017). Screening and Assessment. *British Dyslexia Association*, 8(8). Retrieved from http://www.bdadyslexia.org.uk/educator/ screening-and-assessment

Brousseau-Lachaine, O., Gagnon, F. R., & Faubert, J. (2008). Mild traumatic brain injury induces prolonged visual processing deficits in children. *Brain Injury*, 22(9), 657–668. https://doi.org/10.1080/02699050802203353

Butterworth, B. (2018). Dyscalculia: From science to education. *Science*, 332, 1049–1053. https://doi.org/10.1126/science.1201536

Casey, J. E. (2016). Nonverbal learning disorder: Past, present, and future. In *Special and Gifted Education: Concepts, Methodologies, Tools, and Applications* (pp. 130–168). Hershey, PA: IGI Global.

Chakravarty, A. (2009). Artistic talent in dyslexia—A hypothesis. *Medical Hypotheses*, 73(4), 569–571. https://doi.org/10.1016/j.mehy.2009.05.034

Chideridou–Mandari, A., Padeliadu, S., Karamatsouki, A., Sandravelis, A., & Karagiannidis, C. (2016). Secondary mathematics teachers: What they know and don't know about dyscalculia. *International Journal of Learning, Teaching and Educational Research*, 15(9), 84–98.

Cornoldi, C., Mammarella, I., & Goldenring-Fine, J. (2016). *Nonverbal Learning Disabilities*. New York, London: The Guilford Press.

Cortiella, C., & Horowitz, S. H. (2014). *The State of Learning Disabilities: Facts, Trends and Emerging Issues*. New York: National Center for Learning Disabilities.

Cowan, N. (2008). What are the differences between long-term, short-term, and working memory? *Progress in Brain Research*, 169, 323–338. https://doi. org/10.1016/S0079-6123(07)00020-9

Curatolo, P., D'Agati, E., & Moavero, R. (2010). The neurobiological basis of ADHD. *Italian Journal of Pediatrics*, 36(1), 79. https://doi.org/10.1186/1824-7288-36-79

Dyspraxia Foundation. (2018). What is dyspraxia? Retrieved from https:// dyspraxiafoundation.org.uk/about-dyspraxia/

Franz, C. (2000). Diagnosis and management of nonverbal learning disorders. Paper presented at the Annual Convention of the National Association of School Psychologists, New Orleans, LA. Retrieved from https://eric.ed.gov/

Frith, U. (1985). Beneath the surface of developmental dyslexia. In K. Patterson, J. Marshall, & M. Coltheart (Eds.), *Surface Dyslexia: Neurological and Cognitive Studies of Phonological Reading* (pp. 301–330). Hillsdale, NJ: Lawrence Erlbaum.

Gathercole, S. E., Hitch, G. J., & Martin, A. J. (1997). Phonological short-term memory and new word learning in children. *Developmental Psychology*, 33(6), 966.

Goswami, U. (2008). Reading, dyslexia and the brain. *Educational Research*, 50(2), 135–148. https://doi.org/10.1080/00131880802082625

Holmes, J., Gathercole, S. E., & Dunning, D. L. (2010). Poor working memory: Impact and interventions. *Advances in Child Development and Behavior*, 39, 1–43.

International Dyslexia Organization. (2015). International Dyslexia Organization Fact Sheet. Retrieved from http://eida.org/fact-sheets/

Johnson, K. (2018). Understanding Auditory Processing Disorder. Retrieved from Understood website: https://www.understood.org/en/learning-attention-issues/child-learning-disabilities/auditory-processing-disorder/understanding-auditory-processing-disorder

Kail, R., & Hall, L. (2001). Distinguishing short-term memory from working memory. *Memory and Cognition*, 29(1), 1–9.

Learning Disabilities Association. (2018). Memory. Retrieved from Learning Disabilities Association website: https://ldaamerica.org/types-of-learning-disabilities/memory/

Lingam, R., Hunt, L. P., Golding, J., Jongmans, M. J., & Emond, A. M. (2009). Prevalence of developmental coordination disorder using the DSM-IV at 7 years of age: A UK population-based study. *Pediatrics*, 123(4), 693–700. https://doi.org/10.1542/peds.2008-1770

Lyon, G. R. (1995). Toward a definition of dyslexia. *Annals of Dyslexia*, 45(1), 1–27. https://doi.org/10.1007/BF02648210

Macdonald, S. J. (2010). Towards a social reality of dyslexia. *British Journal of Learning Disabilities*, 38(4), 271–279.

Mayes, S. D., Calhoun, S. L., & Crowell, E. W. (2000). Learning disabilities and ADHD: Overlapping spectrum disorders. *Journal of Learning Disabilities*, 33(5), 417–424.

McCloskey, M., & Rapp, B. (2017). Developmental dysgraphia: An overview and framework for research. *Cognitive Neuropsychology*, 34, 65–82. https://doi.org/10.1080/02643294.2017.1369016

Misra, H., & Aikat, R. (2016). A survey of visual perceptual disorders in typically developing children, and comparison of motor and motor-free visual perceptual training in such children. *Journal of Neurological Disorders*, 4(296). https://doi.org/doi:10.4172/2329-6895.1000296

Molloy, C., Wilson-Ching, M, Anderson, V. A., Roberts, G., Anderson, P. J., & Doyle, L. (2013). Visual processing in adolescents born extremely low birth weight and/or extremely preterm. *Pediatrics*, 132(3), 704–712. https://doi.org/doi:10.1542/peds.2013–0040

Morris, S. (2002). Promoting social skills among students with nonverbal learning disabilities. *Teaching Exceptional Children*, 34(3), 66–70. https://doi.org/10.1177/004005990203400309

Naser, H., Akram, A., Mandana, R., Afsoon, H. M., & Mehdi, A. (2016). An overview of developmental dysgraphia. *The Scientific Journal of Rehabilitation Medicine*, 5(1), 224–234.

National Center for Learning Disabilities. (2005). Executive function fact sheet. *Retrieved*, 8(15). Retrieved from http://www.ldonline.org/article/24880/

National Center for Learning Disabilities. (2019). The state of LD: Identifying struggling students. Retrieved from National Center for Learning Disabilities website: https://www.ncld.org/identifying-struggling-students

National Institute of Neurological Disorders. (2015). Attention Deficit-Hyperactivity Disorder Information Page. Retrieved from National Institute of Neurological Disorders and Stroke website: https://www.ninds.nih.gov/Disorders/All-Disorders/Attention-Deficit-Hyperactivity-Disorder-Information-Page

NICHD. (2017). National Reading Panel. Retrieved from National Institute of Child Health and Human Development website: http://www.nichd.nih.gov/research/supported/Pages/nrp.aspx/

Noorbala, A.-A., & Akhondzadeh, S. (2006). Attention-deficit/hyperactivity disorder: Etiology and pharmacotherapy. *Arch Iran Med*, 9(4), 374–80.

Portwood, M. (2013). *Understanding Developmental Dyspraxia: A Textbook for Students and Professionals*. UK: David Fulton Publishers.

Quillen, T. F., & Gladstone, K. (2008). About dysgraphia. *Nursing*, 38(5), 26. https://doi.org/10.1097/01.NURSE.0000317668.40925.d8

Quinn, P. O., & Madhoo, M. (2014). A review of attention-deficit/hyperactivity disorder in women and girls: Uncovering this hidden diagnosis. *The Primary Care Companion for CNS Disorders*, 16(3). https://doi.org/10.4088/PCC.13r01596

Qureshi, M. N. I., Min, B., Jo, H. J., & Lee, B. (2016). Multiclass classification for the differential diagnosis on the ADHD subtypes using recursive feature elimination and hierarchical extreme learning machine: Structural MRI study. *Plos One*, 11(8). https://doi.org/10.1371/journal.pone.0160697

Richards, R. G. (1999). *The Source for Dyslexia and Dysgraphia*. East Moline, IL: LinguiSystems.

Richardson, A. J., & Ross, A. J. (2000). Fatty acid metabolism in neurodevelopmental disorder: A new perspective on associations between attention-deficit/hyperactivity disorder, dyslexia, dyspraxia and the autistic spectrum. *Prostaglandins Leukotrienes and Essential Fatty Acids*, 63(1), 1–9. https://doi.org/10.1054/plef.2000.0184

Roeser, R., & Downs, M. (2004). *Auditory Disorders in School Children: The Law, Identification, Remediation*. New York: Thieme.

Rosen, P. (2018). Working memory: What it is and how it works. Retrieved from Understood website: https://www.understood.org/en/learning-attention-issues/child-learning-disabilities/executive-functioning-issues/working-memory-what-it-is-and-how-it-works

Semrud-Clikeman, M., Pliszka, S. R., & Liotti, M. (2008). Executive functioning in children with attention-deficit/hyperactivity disorder: Combined type with and without a stimulant medication history. *Neuropsychology (Journal)*, 22(3), 329–340. https://doi.org/10.1037/0894-4105.22.3.329

Shalev, R. (2001). Developmental dyscalculia. *Journal of Child Neurology*, 19(10), 765–771. https://doi.org/10.1177/08830738040190100601

Shaywitz, S. (2003). *Overcoming Dyslexia: A New and Complete Science-Based Program for Reading Problems at Any Level*. USA: Vintage Press.

Skogli, E. W., Teicher, M. H., Andersen, P., Hovik, K. T., & Øie, M. (2013). ADHD in girls and boys – Gender differences in co-existing symptoms and executive function measures. *BMC Psychiatry*, 13(1), 298–298. https://doi.org/i: 10.1186/1471-244X-13-298.

Spreen, O. (2011). Nonverbal learning disabilities: A critical review. *Child Neuropsychology*, 17(5), 418–443. https://doi.org/10.1080/09297049.2010.546778

Sugden, D., Kirby, A., & Dunford, C. (2008). Issues surrounding children with developmental coordination disorder. *International Journal of Disability, Development and Education*, 55(2), 173–187. https://doi.org/doi:10.1080/10349120802033691

Tanaka, H., Black, J. M., Hulme, C., Stanley, L. M., Kesler, S. R., Whitfield-Gabrieli, S., ... Hoeft, F. (2011). The brain basis of the phonological deficit in dyslexia is independent of IQ. *Psychological Science*, 22(11), 1442–1451.

Willcutt, E. G., Doyle, A. E., Nigg, J. T., Faraone, S. V., & Pennington, B. F. (2005). Validity of the executive function theory of attention-deficit/hyperactivity disorder: A meta-analytic review. *Biological Psychiatry*, 57(11), 1336–1346. https://doi.org/10.1016/j.biopsych.2005.02.006

Wilson, A. J., Andrewes, S. G., Struthers, H., Rowe, V. M., Bogdanovic, R., & Waldie, K. E. (2015). Dyscalculia and dyslexia in adults: Cognitive bases of comorbidity. *Learning and Individual Differences*, 37, 118–132. https://doi.org/10.1016/j.lindif.2014.11.017

Zwicker, J., Missiuna, C., Harris, S., & Boyd, L. (2010). Brain activation of children with developmental coordination disorder is different than peers. *Pediatrics*, 126(3), 678–686. https://doi.org/doi:10.1542/peds.2010-0059

6 Working with Students

In this part:

- Background
- Why work with these students?

Background

Elementary school counselors who work with students who have learning disabilities are tasked with an enormous responsibility. The connection between early academic success and later academic success is quite clear (National Center for Learning Disabilities, 2019). Children who struggle with academics early in their school careers without appropriate and viable interventions are at risk for continued academic challenges. Elementary school provides the important basics of literacy and mathematics that continue to build upon themselves all throughout a student's educational life. When these basic skills are not learned early on, students may find it difficult to catch up later and this can lead to continued academic struggles. As elementary school counselors, it is sometimes difficult to see the connection between what happens in elementary school and how that might translate into high school or post high school success, but the connection between them is irrefutable. Unfortunately, many students with learning disabilities are either never identified or are identified too late (National Center for Learning Disabilities, 2019).

The reason so many children are not identified or are identified too late are varied. For example, for many young children signs of possible learning disabilities may manifest as school refusal (National Center for Learning Disabilities, 2019). While the school refusal may be being addressed, the reason behind it as a sign of a potential learning disability may not be. In addition, many parents, scared by the "label" of special education, refuse services even when they are recommended. Additionally, elementary school teachers, who should be the academic front line for identifying these students, do not have the knowledge base to be able to identify a potential learning disability (Nascimento, Rosal, & Queiroga, 2018).

Given the fact that elementary school counselors spend most of their time working on social/emotional issues and parent contact (Perera-Diltz & Mason, 2008), the elementary school counselor is in the perfect position for addressing the issues that may get in the way of identification of learning disabilities. School counselors are the ideal school personnel to address these issues. In addition, school counselors have easy access to all of the players in the identification process: students, teachers, parents and the child study team. Unfortunately, most elementary school counselors are not prepared to work with students with disabilities (Cimsir & Carney, 2017), but it is these students who are in the most dire need.

Why Work with These Students?

Students in elementary school who present with unremediated issues such as social skills deficits, inattention and learning issues are not finding long-term academic success (Rabiner, Godwin, & Dodge, 2016). In addition, the literature is clear in that students with unremediated working memory issues or learning disabilities have a higher likelihood for not attending or dropping out of college (Shapiro et al., 2017), dropping out of high school (Fitzpatrick, Archambault, Janosz, & Pagani, 2015), becoming incarcerated, suffering from depression and/or being unemployed (Cortiella & Horowitz, 2014).

From an academic perspective, teachers working with students with learning disabilities should be teaching using tools such as skills modeling, rehearsal, explicit instruction and frequent feedback (Elias, 2004; Steen & Kaffenberger, 2007), but what about our role as counselors? How can we ensure that we are addressing the needs of these children in a way that can make a significant impact and difference?

COGNITIVE SKILLS TO TEACH STUDENTS

In this part:

- Overview
- Cognitive skills
  - Goal setting
  - Self-efficacy
  - Self-regulation
  - Attending
  - Memory tools

Overview

Current research suggests that there are very specific tools that can be taught to students with learning disabilities in specific and systematic ways. Students with learning disabilities who are taught these skills and are able to implement them have been shown to have better academic outcomes than students who have not been taught these skills (Brigman & Campbell, 2003; Cook et al., 2008; Webb, Brigman, & Campbell, 2005).

In general, these skills can be broken down into two broad categories. The cognitive category encompasses aspects of reasoning and thought, and involves teaching the skills of goal setting, self-efficacy, self-regulation (including metacognition), attending and memory retrieval. The social–emotional category focuses on intrapersonal and interpersonal skills and includes teaching the skills of self-management, self-understanding, resilience, self-advocacy, emotional expression, interpersonal communication, effective listening, teamwork and coping strategies (Brigman & Campbell, 2003; Cleary & Zimmerman, 2004; Cook et al., 2008; Feuerborn & Tyre, 2009; Goddard & Sendi, 2008; Grant & Grant, 2008; Kokkinos & Voulgaridou, 2018; Citro, Michael, & Young, 2018; Webb et al., 2005; Zimmerman, 2000, 2002).

Cognitive Skills

Goal Setting

Goal setting is a cognitive skill that has been shown to have great benefit for students with learning disabilities (Brigman & Campbell, 2003; Cook et al., 2008; Webb et al., 2005). While some students seem to have a natural grasp on this seemingly simple skill, students with learning disabilities seem to struggle with learning how to set goals. The fact that goal setting is really not as simple as it seems to be could certainly be part of the reason for these challenges in learning this skill. Because goal setting is more than just making a statement about what we want to achieve, many students (and adults!) have difficulty understanding how to fit all of the parts of goal setting into their lives. We can say we want to lose ten pounds. We can even dream about losing ten pounds. We can tell everyone we know that we are going to lose ten pounds. The truth is that unless the general goal ("I am going to lose ten pounds") is attached to the specific, measurable, achievable, relevant and time-based steps, or subgoals, necessary to achieve that goal (MacLeod, 2012), then that goal is more wish than potential reality. In order for the sub goals to be meaningful, we have to have certain nuggets of knowledge about both ourselves and the reality that surrounds us. For example, if a subgoal is to stop eating candy from the candy machine at work, then we need to assess the reality of the situation: Are we eating that candy because we aren't organized enough to pack healthy food? If so, the first subgoal should probably be that we pack healthy snacks for work. For our young students with learning disabilities, being able to dissect and understand the steps needed to achieve goals may not be an easy task. Think about what it really takes, for example, to set a goal of reading six chapters of an assigned reading book by the end of the week. First, the student needs to be realistic about their abilities. How much can they actually read in a week? How much can they actually read in a day? Then they have to have an understanding of the level of reading difficulty in the book itself. Is it at a level that they are used to? Is it much easier? Is it much harder? They would also have to be able to make a realistic assessment of what their schedule for the week might look like. Do they have any extracurricular events that week? Are they busy with family activities? Finally, they would have to plan for the unexpected. What course of action is realistic and appropriate, if they find that their plan is not working? For students with learning disabilities, these cognitive paths are not always so clearly defined (Zimmerman, 2002).

Self-Efficacy

Self-efficacy is the belief that students have in their competence and ability as learners (Bandura, 1997). Poor self-efficacy can weaken a student's ability to stay motivated (Bandura, 1997). The belief, based in reality or not, becomes the reality and becomes cyclical failure. A student who believes that they, for example, can't learn math may give up in their efforts to learn the material. This lessened effort might result in less attention paid in class, less time spent on studying and less effort put into assignments. After all, if a student believes that they are not capable of learning, then what is the point of even trying? This behavior leads to poor grades and a continued lack of understanding of the material. As the course progresses and more is taught, the student falls farther and farther behind and the self-fulfilled prophecy of their beliefs about their ability to do math becomes their permanent reality. Bandura (1997) separated the development of self-efficacy beliefs into four main sources. The first source of self-efficacy beliefs is through previous experiences. If a student fails at a particular task, they may begin to feel that they are not capable of doing the task at all. The second source of self-efficacy beliefs can be found in the comparison between self and others. In this instance, if a student sees that many students around them are finding ease in mastering a subject yet they are having difficulty, then they may start to have less of a belief in their ability to master that subject. The third source of self-efficacy comes from the positive or negative persuasion of other people. If a student is surrounded by people who consistently encourage and persuade them that they are capable and good students, then that student may develop a sense of self-efficacy. Finally, the fourth source of self-efficacy is related to the emotional state of the student. If that student feels negative feelings toward the academic task, it can reduce their feelings of self-efficacy. Conversely, by reducing the stress or negative feelings toward the academic task, self-efficacy can still be maintained (Bandura, 1997).

Interestingly, self-esteem, which has for so long been thought to be a component of academic competence, seems to have little to no impact on student achievement (Kokkinos & Voulgaridou, 2018; Ross & Broh, 2000).

Self-Regulation

Self-regulation refers to the skill of being able to monitor one's own learning progress. Although this may seem like a simple task, self-regulation is a complex process that involves the ability to set goals appropriately, have positive motivational beliefs and be able to change course when the learning is not going as planned (Zimmerman, 2002). The process is thought to have four separate components. The first component is described as "forethought" followed by "performance control" and "self-reflection" and finished with "reflection" (Zimmerman, 2000).

Forethought is the first step in the learning process. Forethought is intrinsically tied to the student's beliefs, or self-efficacy, about themselves as learners as well as to goal setting (Cleary & Zimmerman, 2004). So, for example, a student with high levels of self-efficacy, or beliefs about themselves as learners, might approach an assignment or studying for an upcoming test by saying to themselves, "I am going to try to get at least a 95." This learner will then develop a plan of studying or completing the assignment that will help them accomplish this goal. They may decide to study or work on the assignment for 45 minutes every evening until the exam or assignment is due. For this student, their self-efficacy leads them to believe that they are capable of achieving a 95 on the exam. When combined with goal setting, this student is then able to take those beliefs about themselves and translate them into a realistic goal with a viable plan. For a student without this level of self-efficacy, forethought might involve an active decision to disengage from the learning activity. When students have little self-efficacy, or belief in their ability as learners, there is little motivation for engaging in learning activities if they believe that they will not be able to be successful anyway.

The performance control component is based on self-control and self-observation (Zimmerman, 2000). In this cycle, the student is actively engaged in the learning activity. The student may, for example, be actively studying or be actively working on their assignment. In order to be engaged in the learning activity the student has to be engaged in the process of self-control. The student must be able to sustain their attention to the task and the strategies that they have articulated in order to meet their goal. Self-observation, a form of metacognition, is the act of being able to self-monitor performance. A student engaged in the performance control cycle will be actively engaged in the learning activity using self-control to maintain that engagement and will, at the same time, be monitoring their own progress. For example, a student who is engaging in self-observation while studying might keep track of what they have and have not learned yet. They might also be actively asking themselves metacognitive questions such as "Do I really understand this or have I just memorized it?" or "Do I understand this enough or do I need to find another way to study this so I can understand it even more?"

In general, metacognition, although only a small element of self-regulation, is an important element in student achievement. In its most basic form, metacognition is the act of how we think about thinking. For students, metacognitive skills have been shown to have a significant and positive impact on academic success (Wagner & Sternberg, 1984). Because learning is most dynamic when it is meaningful, retained and actively participated in (Hartman, 2001), the act of simply memorizing lists is not enough. In addition to the memorization, metacognition involves thinking about the thinking process as well as the products of those thoughts (Hartman, 2001).

The final component of self-regulation is really viewed as more of the start of the next cycle. This final phase of self-regulation allows the cyclical processes to influence each other and affect future learning. In this phase, the student reflects on their self-regulation process and performance on the test or assignment. The student, upon seeing the end result of their work reflected in the grade they may have earned, decides if they have met their goal and determines how they stand compared to the rest of the class and to themselves. If they have done well, then they can view their strategies as having worked well and can employ them again for the next time. If they have not met their goal or expectations, then the student must make a determination about what needs to be changed or modified in their strategies for future studying. Again, high-achieving students tend to have better metacognitive skills than students who struggle academically (Hartman, 2001; Trainin & Swanson, 2005). In terms of self-regulation, these better metacognitive skills can be seen in the fact that research has shown that students with high grade point averages (GPAs) could more accurately and confidently predict what their grades would be in a given course, whereas students with lower GPAs tended to overestimate their grades (Prohaska, 1994).

An interesting side note to this is the idea of causal attribution (Weiner, 1979). Students who receive a poor grade despite intensive studying may approach the reason for this poor grade in many different ways. Causal attribution refers to what students determine is the cause for a poor grade. For many students, the teacher is to blame. "He didn't teach me this stuff" or "she is a terrible teacher" are the war cries of these students. For other students, their own study habits may be at fault. They may not have studied enough or they may not have studied the correct topics. Students who are able to attribute the cause of their grades to themselves and controllable events (e.g., they needed more sleep the night before the test, they needed to have planned their studying better) tend to have more academic success than students who attribute the cause of their grades to outside, uncontrollable events (e.g., the teaching style of the teacher, the classroom environment) (Weiner, 1979).

Teaching self-regulation techniques to students with learning disabilities seems to have a significant positive impact on these students' willingness to reconnect to their academic assignments (Brigman & Campbell, 2003; Cook et al., 2008; Goddard & Sendi, 2008; Citro et al., 2018; Webb et al., 2005).

Attending

The importance of paying attention to academic tasks and learning is intrinsic to academic achievement (Ek, Westerlund, Holmberg, & Fernell, 2011). Many students with learning disabilities have difficulty sustaining their attention to topics, and students who display these attentional deficits tend to have significant academic issues (Daley & Birchwood, 2010). Some researchers claim that this is because these students have difficulty with processing and retaining information (Grant & Grant, 2008). Other researchers say that the reason many students with learning disabilities have difficulty with sustaining attention is based on their history of poor achievement and negative feelings about their abilities. These feelings can then translate into a disenfranchisement from their work and can then create a cycle of failure (Brigman & Campbell, 2003; Cook et al., 2008; Goddard & Sendi, 2008; Webb et al., 2005).

Regardless of the reason for the inattention, this behavior needs to be addressed early on. Students as early as kindergarten age who have difficulty sustaining attention seem to have significant academic issues later on in their academic careers (Pagani, Fitzpatrick, & Parent, 2012). This early inattention is a predictor to later academic struggle, so addressing these issues early on is important for later academic success.

Studies have indicated that there are several kinds of interventions, outside of, or including, medication, that have proven to be highly effective for helping children attend in classes including neurofeedback, behavior modification and mindfulness training (Beauregard & Lévesque, 2006; Carboni, Roach, & Fredrick, 2013; Hodgson, Hutchinson, & Denson, 2014; Purdie, Hattie, & Carroll, 2002).

Neurofeedback therapy, although not a viable therapy for school counselors to practice, deserves mention based on recent research showing some degree of efficacy, although more studies are needed (Van Doren et al., 2019). It is a therapeutic technique that enhances attention by training the student with attention deficit hyperactivity disorder (ADHD) to control certain brainwave patterns by using electroencephalographic technology. This enhances attention and concentration, providing a physiological means of self-control (Beauregard & Lévesque, 2006).

Behavior modification addresses behaviors through the use of well-known learning techniques such as positive and/or negative reinforcement (Purdie et al., 2002). Behavior modification uses rewards and punishments to help shape and mold behavior. For students struggling with attention issues, a behavior modification strategy would be to give rewards and privileges to the student who displays attentive behavior and take them away from a student who does not.

Finally, mindfulness training has been shown to have positive impact on attention as well (Carboni et al., 2013) and has been shown to be effective with young children (Rani & Rao, 1996). Mindfulness is a form of attention that includes intentionality, focus on the present moment, and acceptance of the moment and the thoughts occurring in a nonjudgmental manner (Semple & Lee, 2008). It can be viewed as a form of attention training (Burke, 2010) and is not, as sometimes believed, about emptying all thought out of the mind. It is, rather, about being aware and in the moment (Siegel, Germer, & Cole, 2009). Mindfulness is about being in the present and in the moment and attending to the present moment in a nonjudgmental way (Marlatt & Kristeller, 1999) and directs attention toward something specific such as breath or sound (Semple & Lee, 2008).

Memory

It is clear that memory deficits, especially working memory, can play a significant role in young children's ability to learn and to retain knowledge (Alloway & Gathercole, 2006) and that early working memory issues can predict later academic issues (Fitzpatrick et al., 2015). Young children with working memory deficits have difficulty storing information that they need to use for tasks that need to be engaged in at the moment. Remembering a phone number in order to dial it and then complete a phone call is an example of the use of working memory. A young student with working memory deficits may have difficulty listening for directions and remembering the information that they are being given to work with all at the same time. These children may have difficulty in following multistep directions or following directions in order and these memory issues can then transition into what seem to be attentional issues. Imagine, for example, that you have a long list of things to do and as you begin to do them, you forget what you are even doing in the room you are standing in. Children and adults with working memory issues live in a constant state of this forgetfulness. This translates into a significant amount of mental energy being spent on trying to remember what to do next. In terms of learning to read, this focus on remembering precludes the fluency that children are expected to achieve. If you are always trying to remember what the letter "A" sounds like, it becomes that much more difficult to learn to read with fluency. In terms of math, since math is linear and builds upon itself, one misstep early in the math problem can lead to the wrong answer. For students with memory issues, these missteps can be constant and can interfere with learning the sequence that math is made of. Improvements in working memory can improve the ability to problem-solve. This can translate into better academics as well as better social skills (McQuade, Murray-Close, Shoulberg, & Hoza, 2013).

When working with students to help them with memory issues, there are multiple training methods that seem to have some degree of efficacy.

1. Repeated practice: Students who practice their learning and slowly increase the challenges, in conjunction with addressing social/ emotional skills, seem to have success in increasing memory retention (Diamond & Lee, 2011).

2. Gesturing: Students who use gestures in addition to, or in order to, recall learning have a significant higher rate of recall than those who don't (Stevanoni & Salmon, 2005). One reason that gesturing may be helpful in recall is that it becomes a cue for items that have been learned. Attaching the gesture to the learning creates a milieu where the gesture becomes the cue for the information needed to be recalled. Another explanation for its efficacy could be that the gesture becomes a vehicle for holding onto the cognitive bundle that would otherwise become working memory. For students with working memory deficits, storing the information inside the gesture might take the load off of working memory (Stevanoni & Salmon, 2005). A final explanation for this higher rate of recall through gesturing is that the physical action of the gesture itself might be the agent that increases engagement in the learning and thus allows for better recall (Stevanoni & Salmon, 2005).

3. Mnemonics: Researchers have long concluded that mnemonic training is helpful to students with learning disabilities (Hampstead, Sathian, Bikson, & Stringer, 2017; Simon et al., 2018). Mnemonics are strategies that are designed to help people remember new information. They act as linguistic, visual, spatial, verbal or physical links to prior information that make retrieval of new information and concepts more accessible (Thompson, 1987).

    Linguistic mnemonics associate the new learning with phrases or words. This type of mnemonic can be used in multiple ways. Acronyms, for example, are words or phrases formed from the first letter of each word in a list of words. "ROY G BIV," for example, is an acronym used to remember the order of and the colors of the rainbow. Each letter stands for each successive color in the rainbow – red, orange, yellow, green, blue, indigo and violet.

    Visual mnemonics uses pictures or even mental visualizations to create connections to the new learning. In order for a student to remember, for example, that Isaac Newton is connected to the laws of gravity, the student might visualize Isaac Newton falling from the sky. This visualization would solidify the connection between Isaac Newton and his connection to the laws of gravity.

    Spatial mnemonics use familiar spaces or patterns to create connections to the new learning. The memorization technique known as the method of the loci, which requires students to mentally place items that they are required to remember into a mental image of a place they are completely familiar with, is a form of spatial mnemonics.

Verbal mnemonics uses meaningful stories to help students make the connections to new knowledge. This type of mnemonic uses storytelling or narratives to remember the new information. For example, if a student is asked to remember the order of biological classification, which is kingdom, phylum, class, order, family, genus and species, a student might create a story that might look like this:

> Once upon a time there was a KINGDOM which was ruled by the mighty king PHYLUM. When King Phylum was a boy, he was a very good student in all of his subjects but his favorite CLASS was math. He liked math the best because numbers always came in the same ORDER and that made it easy to remember. His FAMILY was very proud of him, especially his very smart uncle who they called uncle GENUS. King Phylum's whole family joked that his math abilities were so unique in their family that even though he was obviously a member of their family, he must have come from a whole different SPECIES.

Since it may be easier to remember this silly story than the list of words that make up the list of biological classifications, using this verbal mnemonic may be more useful in remembering the words and their order than in just trying to memorize them.

Physical mnemonics use movement or sensation to create connections to new learning. Students attach a movement to the new learning to be remembered. For example, a student learning a new math fact may be asked to jump up and down three times during the learning in order to concretize the connection to the new learning.

4. Integrative elaboration: Integrative elaboration involves activation prior knowledge in a discussion format in order to solidify new learning (Arbuthnott & Krätzig, 2015). This kind of discussion prior to study session can make the newly learned material more meaningful and therefore easier to retrieve.

5. Retrieval practice: Retrieval practice is simply the act of bringing the newly learned information into focus frequently (Hascher, 2010). On a very simplistic and daily level, a young child who is learning how to tie their own shoes will solidify this learning much more quickly if they practice this skill frequently. In educational settings, frequent testing, whether it is self-testing as a study method or teacher driven testing, is found to have the same effect (Arbuthnott & Krätzig, 2015).

6. Distributed learning: Distributed learning is done when the instruction is spread and practiced over time so that the knowledge gets repeated frequently (Arbuthnott & Krätzig, 2015).

7. Coping strategies: Children who learn how to deal with stress by using specifically taught coping strategies tend to have less memory issues than children who do not use these skills (Vogel & Schwabe, 2016). Good coping strategies could include the following:

   Deep breathing: Teaching students deep breathing strategies as a tool for coping and stress relief has been shown to be extremely efficacious (Paul, Elam, & Verhulst, 2007).

   Labeling feelings: Students who learn how to name their feelings appropriately seem to be able to resolve problems better, make friends more easily and manage their environments in a much more positive way than children who do not know how to name their feelings appropriately (Hansen & Zambo, 2007; Mun, 2008).

   Exercise: Students who participate in physical activity seem to show improvement in their coping strategies as well as their perceived levels of stress (Kantomaa, Tammelin, Ebeling, & Taanila, 2008; Oddie et al., 2014).

   Positive self-talk: Positive self-talk has been related to better academic performance. Both instructional self-talk (telling oneself how to accomplish a task) and motivational self-talk (giving oneself encouragement) have been shown to work together to increase academic performance (Sanchez & Carvajal, 2016).

8. Emotional learning: Emotional learning is based on the concept that children remember learned material better when an emotional component is infused into the learning (Vogel & Schwabe, 2016). For example, children who feel respected for their early learning attempts tend to associate these positive feelings with later learning as well (Hascher, 2010). Likewise, teachers who enjoy teaching and therefore tend to be more creative and supporting during students' learning seem to have students who achieve higher than the students of teachers who don't seem to enjoy teaching as much (Valeski & Stipek, 2001). This emotional component on the teachers' end creates a culture of positivity and acceptance and therefore can have a positive impact on later student motivation to learn (Krapp, 2002; Valeski & Stipek, 2001).

9. Memory training programs: It should be noted that working memory training programs, such as Cogmed, have been widely used. Although these types of memory training programs may actually help temporarily by improving some aspects of short-term memory, these programs have not been proven to be completely efficacious and do not seem to transfer into long-term memory. The results of the research are inconsistent and fairly mixed (Kroesbergen, van't Noordende, & Kolkman, 2014). The recommendations for this kind of training, given the cost, the loss of learning time and the lack of transfer to long term memory, are not positive (Roberts et al., 2016).

SOCIAL–EMOTIONAL SKILLS TO TEACH STUDENTS

In this part:

- Social–emotional skills
  - Self-management
  - Self-understanding
  - Resilience
  - Self-advocacy
  - Emotional expression
  - Social skills
  - Coping techniques

Social–Emotional Skills

Self-Management

Self-management skills include the ability to manage attention, anger and motivation. The ability to self-manage these three areas is highly correlated to long-term school success and seems to be the mitigating factor in the difference between high achievers and low achievers (Brigman & Campbell, 2003; Webb et al., 2005).

Self-management includes the ability to manage attention. Being able to manage attention is a significant part of academic success (Ek et al., 2011). Students with learning disabilities tend to have difficulty keeping their attention on academic topics, and this lack of attention can lead to serious learning deficits and academic issues (Daley & Birchwood, 2010). Regardless of the reason for this lack of attention, this behavior can create a cycle of failure and academic disengagement (Brigman & Campbell, 2003; Cook et al., 2008; Goddard & Sendi, 2008; Webb et al., 2005). It is important to note that early intervention with attentional issues can have significant positive impact on later academic achievement (Pagani et al., 2012). Both behavior modification and mindfulness training have been shown to have great positive impact on dealing with attentional issues (Carboni et al., 2013; Purdie et al., 2002). Behavior modification uses a combination of punishment and reward to create the desired behavior, while mindfulness training helps the student stay connected to the present moment to be aware of behavior as it occurs (Semple & Lee, 2008).

Another aspect of self-management is the ability to manage anger. Although anger is a normal reaction to some situations, it does need to be held in check and regulated. Students can be taught how to respond to their feeling of anger to keep themselves from either blowing up at others or internalizing it (Merrell, 2013).

One last part of self-management involves managing motivation. Motivation is intrinsically tied into student academic success, but students are reluctant to be motivated to accomplish a task if they don't know or don't understand the value inherent in the task (Zimmerman, 2000). It seems that the students with learning disabilities who continue to experience failure seem to experience more hopelessness, negative emotions and a lack of motivation than other students who don't experience failure (Boekaerts, De Koning, & Vedder, 2006; Sideridis, 2003). Interestingly, these students seem to lose motivation when teachers seem to value grades over personal improvement and, conversely, seem to thrive when teachers value personal improvement over grades (Sideridis, 2003).

Self-Understanding

The ability to understand oneself, both as a learner and as a whole person, is pivotal to student success (Citro et al., 2018). One major aspect of self-understanding that relates directly to students with individualized education plans (IEPs) is based on the students' abilities to read and understand their IEPs. The earlier students are able to understand and feel positive towards their IEPs, including understanding what their strengths and challenges are, the higher the likelihood of these students achieving academic success (Rothman & Cosden, 1995). In order for students to understand their learning needs, they need to be able to understand themselves as learners first (Test, Fowler, Wood, Brewer, & Eddy, 2005). These students need to be able to understand and talk about their learning disability. For many students, all they know is that they might have trouble with reading or math. They may not know that they have a learning disability. They may not know that having a learning disability does not correlate with a lack of intelligence. They may not know how smart they really are.

Resilience

Resilience can be separated into cognitive resilience and social–emotional resilience. Cognitive resilience refers to the ability of students with learning disabilities to continue to attempt to acquire academic skills even if the skills are difficult (Haft, Myers, & Hoeft, 2016). Social–emotional resilience refers to the ability to overcome interpersonal or intrapersonal problems. Students with learning disabilities who are able to "bounce back" from adversity, frustration and failure are far more likely to have better academic outcomes than students who do not possess these skills (Citro et al., 2018; Haft et al., 2016).

Self-Advocacy

Self-advocacy involves the skill of being able to advocate for needs appropriately and is a skill that is integral to the success of students with learning disabilities (Citro et al., 2018). Most children, especially young children, do not know how to advocate for themselves. As counselors, we can work with these children and teach them these skills and strategies so that they can learn to advocate for themselves. For students with learning disabilities, learning these self-advocacy skills early on can become the difference between success and failure. Self-advocacy skills have been shown to have a significant and positive effect on college retention (Field, Sarver, & Shaw, 2003) and children who have these skills are more likely to be successful later on in school than students who have not been taught these skills (Field et al., 2003). These skills are specific and teachable (Arkeny & Lehmann, 2010) and are specifically tied into learning disabilities.

Emotional Expression

Students with learning disabilities may have challenges in recognizing and naming their emotions (Elias, 2004). This inability to understand their own emotions is tied to both academic and social challenges (Citro et al., 2018). These students can be taught skills and vocabulary to help them become more emotionally connected to themselves. For example, counselors can teach students "I feel …" statements. For example, if a student is having a confrontation with another student who has said something mean to them, the student can be taught to say, "I feel upset when you say mean things to me" (Feuerborn & Tyre, 2009).

Social Skills

Social skills deficits seem to be directly connected to learning disabilities (Barber & Mueller, 2011). Students with learning disabilities seem to have issues with interpersonal skills, social problem-solving, listening and teamwork skills (Brigman & Campbell, 2003; Webb et al., 2005). Despite the fact that there are a number of social skills training programs available, the research does not substantiate social skills training as an efficacious method of managing social skills issues (Kavale & Forness, 1996; Kavale & Mostert, 2004). Instead of targeted social skills training, what has been found to have significant impact in all areas is the implementation of social/emotional learning programs (Elias, 2004; Espelage, Rose, & Polanin, 2016).

Coping Techniques

Implementing coping techniques gives students the vehicle they need to work through difficult situations (Feuerborn & Tyre, 2009). Counselors can teach students coping techniques such as how to identify physical cues to understand feelings of stress, deep breathing, progressive relaxation, positive self-talk and mindfulness.

BEST PRACTICES IN TEACHING THE SKILLS

In order to best teach the cognitive and social–emotional skills that work best to help our students to succeed, the literature is very clear about how best to approach it. There are several very specific methods of teaching these skills.

The first thing to keep in mind for teaching these skills to is keep the groups small and structured. A small and structured group format with ten students or less seems to work best for teaching these kinds of skills (Webb et al., 2005). The small group allows students to maintain direct contact with the group facilitator at all time while the structured format ensures that the specific skills that are to be taught actually get taught.

The structure that seems to work best for these kinds of groups is a structure that uses the "ask, tell, show, do, and feedback" loop (Brigman & Campbell, 2003; Webb et al., 2005). What this means is that the counselor/facilitator begins the session by asking questions about the skill. The counselor or facilitator then tells the students what the skill is and then follows this with showing the students what the skill actually looks like. The group finishes with having the students practice the skill in the group and are then given constructive feedback.

Peer modeling has also been shown to be an excellent method of learning these skills (Trusty, Mellin, & Herbert, 2008). Within the small group and the structured format, peer modeling of appropriate skills allows students who may still be shaky in those areas to observe peer models.

References

Alloway, T. P., & Gathercole, S. E. (2006). *Working Memory and Neurodevelopmental Disorders*. New York: Psychology Press.

Arbuthnott, K. D., & Krätzig, G. P. (2015). Effective teaching: Sensory learning styles versus general memory processes. *Comprehensive Psychology*, 4, 1–9. https://doi.org/10.2466/06.IT.4.2

Arkeny, E., & Lehmann, J. (2010). Journey toward self-determination: Voices of students with disabilities who participated in a secondary transition program on a community college campus. *Remedial and Special Education*, 32(4), 279–289. https://doi.org/10.1177/0741932510362215

Bandura, A. (1997). *Self-Efficacy: The Exercise of Control*. New York: Freeman.

Barber, C., & Mueller, C. T. (2011). Social and self-perceptions of adolescents identified as gifted, learning disabled, and twice-exceptional. *Roeper Review*, 33(2), 109–120. https://doi.org/10.1080/02783193.2011.554158

Beauregard, M., & Lévesque, J. (2006). Functional magnetic resonance imaging investigation of the effects of neurofeedback training on the neural bases of selective attention and response inhibition in children with attention-deficit/hyperactivity disorder. *Applied Psychophysiology and Biofeedback*, 31(1), 3–20.

Boekaerts, M., De Koning, E., & Vedder, P. (2006). Goal-directed behavior and contextual factors in the classroom: An innovative approach to the study of multiple goals. *Educational Psychologist*, 41(1), 33–51. https://doi.org/10.1207/s15326985ep4101_5

Brigman, G., & Campbell, C. (2003). Helping students improve academic achievement and school success behavior. *Professional School Counseling*, 7(2), 91–98.

Burke, C. A. (2010). Mindfulness-based approaches with children and adolescents: A preliminary review of current research in an emergent field. *Journal of Child and Family Studies*, 19(2), 133–144.

Carboni, J., Roach, A., & Fredrick, L. (2013). Impact of mindfulness training on the behavior of elementary students with attention-deficit/hyperactive disorder. *Research in Human Development*, 10(3), 234–251. https://doi.org/10. 1080/15427609.2013.818487

Cimsir, E., & Carney, J. V. (2017). School counsellor training, attitudes, and perceptions of preparedness to provide services to students with disabilities in inclusive schools in Turkey. *European Journal of Special Needs Education*, 32(3), 346–361. https://doi.org/10.1080/08856257.2016.1240340

Citro, T., Michael, C., & Young, N. (2018). *Emotions and Education: Promoting Positive Mental Health in Students with Learning Disabilities*. Wilmington, DE: Vernon Press.

Cleary, T. J., & Zimmerman, B. J. (2004). Self-regulation empowerment program: A school-based program to enhance self-regulated and self-motivated cycles of student learning. *Psychology in the Schools*, 41(5), 537–550. https://doi. org/10.1002/pits.10177

Cook, C. R., Gresham, F. M., Kern, L., Barreras, R. B., Thornton, S., & Crews, S. D. (2008). Social skills training for secondary students with emotional and/ or behavioral disorders: A review and analysis of the meta-analytic literature. *Journal of Emotional and Behavioral Disorders*, 16(3), 131–144. https://doi. org/10.1177/1063426608314541

Cortiella, C., & Horowitz, S. H. (2014). *The State of Learning Disabilities: Facts, Trends and Emerging Issues*. New York: National Center for Learning Disabilities.

Daley, D., & Birchwood, J. (2010). ADHD and academic performance: Why does ADHD impact on academic performance and what can be done to support ADHD children in the classroom? *Child: Care, Health and Development*, 36(4), 455–464. https://doi.org/10.1111/j.1365-2214.2009.01046.x

Diamond, A., & Lee, K. (2011). Interventions shown to aid executive function development in children 4 to 12 years old. *Science*, 333(6045), 959–964. https:// doi.org/10.1126/science.1204529

Ek, U., Westerlund, J., Holmberg, K., & Fernell, E. (2011). Academic performance of adolescents with ADHD and other behavioural and learning problems—A population-based longitudinal study. *Acta Paediatrica*, 100(3), 402–406. https:// doi.org/10.1111/j.1651-2227.2010.02048.x

Elias, M. J. (2004). The connection between social-emotional learning and learning disabilities: Implications for intervention. *Learning Disability Quarterly*, 27(1), 53–63. https://doi.org/10.2307/1593632

Espelage, D. L., Rose, C. A., & Polanin, J. R. (2016). Social-emotional learning program to promote prosocial and academic skills among middle school students with disabilities. *Remedial and Special Education*, 37(6), 323–332. https://doi.org/10.1177/0741932515627475

Feuerborn, L., & Tyre, A. (2009). Practical social-emotional learning tools for students with specific learning disabilities in the United States of America. *Journal of the International Association of Special Education*, 10(1), 21–25.

Field, S., Sarver, M. D., & Shaw, S. F. (2003). Self-determination: A key to success in postsecondary education for students with learning disabilities. *Remedial and Special Education*, 24, 339–349. https://doi.org/0.1177/07419325030240060501

Fitzpatrick, C., Archambault, I., Janosz, M., & Pagani, L. S. (2015). Early childhood working memory forecasts high school dropout risk. *Intelligence*, 53, 160–165. https://doi.org/10.1016/j.intell.2015.10.002

Goddard, Y., & Sendi, C. (2008). Effects of self-monitoring on the narrative and expository writing of four fourth-grade students with learning disabilities. *Reading & Writing Quarterly*, 24(4), 408–433. https://doi.org/10.1080/10573560802004514

Grant, P., & Grant, P. (2008). Educating children with specific learning disabilities. In P. Peterson (Ed.), *International Encyclopedia of Education* (3rd ed., pp. 646–653). Philadelphia, PA: Elsevier.

Haft, S. L., Myers, C. A., & Hoeft, F. (2016). Socio-emotional and cognitive resilience in children with reading disabilities. *Current Opinion in Behavioral Sciences*, 10, 133–141. https://doi.org/10.1016/j.cobeha.2016.06.005

Hampstead, B. M., Sathian, K., Bikson, M., & Stringer, A. Y. (2017). Combined mnemonic strategy training and high-definition transcranial direct current stimulation for memory deficits in mild cognitive impairment. *Alzheimer's & Dementia: Translational Research & Clinical Interventions*, 3(3), 459–470.

Hansen, C. C., & Zambo, D. (2007). Loving and learning with Wemberly and David: Fostering emotional development in early childhood education. *Early Childhood Education Journal*, 34(4), 273–278.

Hartman, H. (2001). Developing students' metacognitive knowledge and skills. In H. Hartman (Ed.), *Metacognition in Learning and Instruction* (pp. 33–68). Netherlands: Springer.

Hascher, T. (2010). Learning and emotion: Perspectives for theory and research. *European Educational Research Journal*, 9(1), 13–28. https://doi.org/10.2304/eerj.2010.9.1.13

Hodgson, K., Hutchinson, A. D., & Denson, L. (2014). Nonpharmacological treatments for ADHD: A meta-analytic review. *Journal of Attention Disorders*, 18(4), 275–282. https://doi.org/10.1177/1087054712444732

Kantomaa, M. T., Tammelin, T. H., Ebeling, H. E., & Taanila, A. M. (2008). Emotional and behavioral problems in relation to physical activity in youth. *Medicine and Science in Sports and Exercise*, 40(10), 1749–1756. https://doi.org/10.1249/MSS.0b013e31817b8e82

Kavale, K. A., & Forness, S. R. (1996). Social skill deficits and learning disabilities: A meta-analysis. *Journal of Learning Disabilities*, 29(3), 226–237. https://doi.org/10.1177/002221949602900301

Kavale, K. A., & Mostert, M. P. (2004). Social skills interventions for individuals with learning disabilities. *Learning Disability Quarterly*, 27(1), 31–43. https://doi.org/10.2307/1593630

Kokkinos, C. M., & Voulgaridou, I. (2018). Motivational beliefs as mediators in the association between perceived scholastic competence, self-esteem and learning strategies among Greek secondary school students. *Educational Psychology*, 38(6), 753–771. https://doi.org/10.1080/01443410.2018.1456651

Krapp, A. (2002). Structural and dynamic aspects of interest development: Theoretical considerations from an ontogenetic perspective. *Learning and Instruction*, 12(4), 383–409. https://doi.org/10.1016/S0959-4752(01)00011-1

Kroesbergen, E. H., van't Noordende, J. E., & Kolkman, M. E. (2014). Training working memory in kindergarten children: Effects on working memory and early numeracy. *Child Neuropsychology*, 20(1), 23–37. https://doi.org/10.1080/09297049.2012.736483

MacLeod, L. (2012). Making SMART goals smarter. *Physician Executive*, 38(2), 68–72.

Marlatt, G., & Kristeller, J. (1999). Mindfulness and meditation. In W. Miller (Ed.), *Integrating Spirituality into Treatment* (pp. 67–84). Washington, DC: American Psychological Association.

McQuade, J. D., Murray-Close, D., Shoulberg, E. K., & Hoza, B. (2013). Working memory and social functioning in children. *Journal of Experimental Child Psychology*, 115(3), 422–435. https://doi.org/10.1016/j.jecp.2013.03.002

Merrell, K. W. (2013). *Helping Students Overcome Depression and Anxiety: A Practical Guide*. New York: Guilford Publications.

Mun, W. (2008). Helping young children to develop adaptive coping strategies. *Journal of Basic Education*, 17(1).

Nascimento, I. S. do, Rosal, A. G. C., & Queiroga, B. A. M. de. (2018). Elementary school teachers' knowledge on dyslexia. *Revista CEFAC*, 20(1), 87–94. http://dx.doi.org/10.1590/1982-021620182019117

National Center for Learning Disabilities. (2019). The state of LD: Identifying struggling students. Retrieved from National Center for Learning Disabilities website: https://www.ncld.org/identifying-struggling-students

Oddie, S., Fredeen, D., Williamson, B., DeClerck, D., Doe, S., & Moslenko, K. (2014). Can physical activity improve depression, coping and motivation to exercise in children and youth experiencing challenges to mental wellness? *Psychology*, 5(19), 2147. https://doi.org/10.4236/psych.2014.519217

Pagani, L., Fitzpatrick, C., & Parent, S. (2012). Relating kindergarten attention to subsequent developmental pathways of classroom engagement in elementary school. *Journal of Abnormal Child Psychology*, 40(5), 715–725. https://doi.org/10.1007/s10802-011-9605-4

Paul, G., Elam, B., & Verhulst, S. J. (2007). A longitudinal study of students' perceptions of using deep breathing meditation to reduce testing stresses. *Teaching and Learning in Medicine*, 19(3), 287–292. https://doi.org/10.1080/10401330701366754

Perera-Diltz, D. M., & Mason, K. L. (2008). Ideal to real: Duties performed by school counselors. *Journal of School Counseling*, 6(26), n26.

Prohaska, V. (1994). "I know I'll get an A": Confident overestimation of final course grades. *Teaching of Psychology*, 21(3), 141–143. https://doi.org/10.1177/009862839402100303

Purdie, N., Hattie, J., & Carroll, A. (2002). A review of the research on interventions for attention deficit hyperactivity disorder: What works best? *Review of Educational Research*, 72(1), 61–99. https://doi.org/10.3102/00346543072001061

Rabiner, D. L., Godwin, J., & Dodge, K. A. (2016). Predicting academic achievement and attainment: The contribution of early academic skills, attention difficulties, and social competence. *School Psychology Review*, 45(2), 250–267.

Rani, N., & Rao, P. (1996). Meditation and attention regulation. *Journal of Indian Psychology*, 14(1–2), 26–30.

Roberts, G., Quach, J., Spencer-Smith, M., Anderson, P. J., Gathercole, S., Gold, L., … Ainley, J. (2016). Academic outcomes 2 years after working memory training for children with low working memory: A randomized clinical trial. *JAMA Pediatrics*, 170(5), 1–10. https://doi.org/10.1001/jamapediatrics.2015.4568

Ross, C. E., & Broh, B. A. (2000). The roles of self-esteem and the sense of personal control in the academic achievement process. *Sociology of Education*, 73(4), 270–284. https://doi.org/10.2307/2673234

Rothman, H. R., & Cosden, M. (1995). The relationship between self-perception of a learning disability and achievement, self-concept and social support. *Learning Disability Quarterly*, 18(3), 203–212. https://doi.org/10.2307/1511043

Sanchez, F., & Carvajal, F. (2016). Self-talk and academic performance in undergraduate students. *Anales de Psicología*, 32(1), 139. http://dx.doi.org/10.6018/analesps.32.1.188441

Semple, R., & Lee, J. (2008). Treating anxiety with mindfulness: Mindfulness-based cognitive therapy for children. In L. Greco & S. Hayes (Eds.), *Acceptance and Mindfulness Treatments for Children and Adolescents: A Practitioner's Guide*. Oakland, CA: New Harbinger Publication, Inc.

Shapiro, D., Dundar, A., Huie, F., Wakhungu, P. K., Yuan, X., Nathan, A., & Bhimdiwali, A. (2017). Completing college: A national view of student completion rates–Fall 2011 cohort. Retrieved from National Student Clearinghouse Research Center website: https://nscresearchcenter.org/signaturereport14/

Sideridis, G. D. (2003). On the origins of helpless behavior of students with learning disabilities: Avoidance motivation? *International Journal of Educational Research*, 39(4–5), 497–517. https://doi.org/10.1016/j.ijer.2004.06.011

Siegel, R., Germer, C., & Cole, C. (2009). Mindfulness: What is it? Where did it come from? In J. Kabat-Zinn (Ed.), *Clinical Handbook of Mindfulness* (pp. 17–35). New York: Springer.

Simon, S. S., Hampstead, B. M., P Nucci, M., Souza-Duran, F. L., M Fonseca, L., Martin, M. da G. M, … Brucki, D. (2018). Cognitive and brain activity changes after mnemonic strategy training in amnestic mild cognitive impairment: Evidence from a randomized controlled trial. *Frontiers in Aging Neuroscience*, 10, 342. https://doi.org/10.3389/fnagi.2018.00342

Steen, S., & Kaffenberger, C. J. (2007). Integrating academic interventions into small group counseling in elementary school. *Professional School Counseling*, 10(5). https://doi.org/10.1177/2156759X0701000510

Stevanoni, E., & Salmon, K. (2005). Giving memory a hand: Instructing children to gesture enhances their event recall. *Journal of Nonverbal Behavior*, 29(4), 217–233.

Test, D. W., Fowler, C. H., Wood, W. M., Brewer, D. M., & Eddy, S. (2005). A conceptual framework of self-advocacy for students with disabilities. *Remedial and Special Education*, 26(1), 43–54.

Thompson, I. (1987). Memory in language learning. In A. Wenden, & J. Rubin (Eds.), *Learner Strategies in Language Learning* (pp. 15–30). Englewood Cliffs, NJ: Prentice Hall.

Trainin, G., & Swanson, H. L. (2005). Cognition, metacognition, and achievement of college students with learning disabilities. *Learning Disability Quarterly*, 28(4), 261–272. https://doi.org/10.2307/4126965

Trusty, J., Mellin, E. A., & Herbert, J. T. (2008). Closing achievement gaps: Roles and tasks of elementary school counselors. *The Elementary School Journal*, 108(5), 407–421. https://doi.org/10.1086/589470

Valeski, T. N., & Stipek, D. J. (2001). Young children's feelings about school. *Child Development*, 72(4), 1198–1213. https://doi.org/10.1111/1467-8624.00342

Van Doren, J., Arns, M., Heinrich, H., Vollebregt, M. A., Strehl, U., & Loo, S. K. (2019). Sustained effects of neurofeedback in ADHD: a systematic review and meta-analysis. *European Child & Adolescent Psychiatry*, 28(3), 293–305.

Vogel, S., & Schwabe, L. (2016). Learning and memory under stress: Implications for the classroom. *NPJ Science of Learning*, 1. https://doi.org/16011; doi:10.1038/npjscilearn.2016.11

Wagner, R. K., & Sternberg, R. J. (1984). Alternative conceptions of intelligence and their implications for education. *Review of Educational Research*, 54(2), 179–223. https://doi.org/10.3102/00346543054002179

Webb, L. D., Brigman, G. A., & Campbell, C. (2005). Linking school counselors and student success: A replication of the Student Success Skills approach targeting the academic and social competence of students. *Professional School Counseling*, 8(5), 407–413.

Weiner, B. (1979). A theory of motivation for some classroom experiences. *Journal of Educational Psychology*, 71(1), 3.

Zimmerman, B. (2000). Attaining self-regulation: A social-cognitive perspective. In M. Boekaerts, P. Pintrich, & M. Seidner (Eds.), *Self-Regulation: Theory, Research, and Applications* (pp. 13–39). Orlando, FL: Academic Press.

Zimmerman, B. (2002). Achieving self-regulation: The trial and triumph of adolescence. In T. Urdan & F. Pajares (Eds.), *Academic Motivation of Adolescents* (Vol. 2, pp. 1–27). Greenwich, CT: Information Age.

7 Working with the Child Study Team

In this part:

- Child study team (or IEP team)
- IEP meetings
- Relationship with child study team
- Identification

Child Study Team (or IEP Team)

In order for a school system to determine if a child has a specific learning disability and is considered disabled as defined by the U.S. government, a team of qualified professionals must make that determination together. According to the law, that team needs to be comprised of the child's parent, the child's general education teacher and at least one person who is credentialed to conduct a diagnostic examination. This person is typically a school psychologist, speech-language pathologist or remedial reading teacher (Individuals with Disabilities Education Act [IDEA], 1997).

In my district, our child study team consists of a school social worker, a learning consultant and a school psychologist. Our students with learning disabilities have the wonderful advantage of having multiple supports and advocates within their school day. They have us, their school counselors, but they are also assigned a member of the child study team as a case manager and also have the entire child study team standing behind them as well. These members of the child study team work together to identify, evaluate, place and case-manage students with disabilities. These are the professionals who are tasked with writing and overseeing implementation of the individualized education plans (IEPs) for all students who are classified as having disabilities within the school. Their job is to create the most appropriate educational program for these students while still staying within the boundaries of the law and district budgets, and this is certainly no small task. There are timelines that need to be adhered to, reports that need to be written and meetings that have to be held and all of this has to be done within a specific framework of time. These are the professionals who are the most familiar with the special education system and they are the crux of the academic process for students with disabilities.

IEP Meetings

IEP meetings are held for a number of different reasons. An IEP meeting is held after a child is found eligible for special education in order to determine placement. In addition, IEP meetings are held at least annually in order to review the progress that a student has made and make any necessary programming updates. Every IEP meeting must include specific information including present performance, goals, and objectives, and a description of the services that will be provided to the student. For students who are already classified, a reevaluation must be conducted every three years. If testing has been readministered for this student (which may not need to be done if a functional assessment is used instead), the results of the reevaluation are discussed as well. Attendance at IEP meetings is mandatory for certain people and there are guidelines about who must attend, but generally, an IEP meeting will involve the parent, the child (if it is determined that attendance is in the best interest of the child), a general education teacher, a special education teacher and a member of the child study team.

Since counselors have a very unique position in a school setting, it is important that the counselor attend IEP meetings. As you can see from the guidelines, counselors are not mandated by law to attend IEP meetings but since counselors are the people who can truly and impartially advocate for our students (Erford & Erford, 2007), it makes sense that we attend these meetings.

We can be there because the meeting gives us a venue for collaboration and dialogue. It is important for everyone to work together to help our students succeed and these invitations to have a seat at the table provide those opportunities. School counselors and child study teams seem to continue to live on separate islands and our input rounds out whatever other information is available about the child. The classroom teachers may only have a view of the student based on their classroom performance and behavior, child study team members may only be focused on the special education aspect of the meeting, and administrators (if they are present) may not know the student at all.

As counselors, we are trained to see a wholistic picture of the child and that ability makes us that impartial advocate that the student may need. As counselors, we may have specialized insight into all of the factors that may be having an impact on the success of a student. The counselor may know, for example, that the reason the student may not be handing in homework is because this student's home situation may preclude their ability to do the work. The counselor then becomes an invaluable source of information in deciding the best programing route for the student. It is important to remember that just attending the IEP meeting is not enough. Counselors should not just be silently sitting back in the meeting and listening. The contributions that we are able to provide through our unique perspectives as counselors can enhance the entire structure of the IEP meeting itself.

There is valuable insight about the student to be gained from sitting in on IEP meeting. There are too few times in a student's education that so many important stakeholders get to sit around a table and discuss the student in detail. The IEP meeting is an opportunity for us to hear all of the different views about the student's progress and it gives us an opportunity to explore what might otherwise be gaps in information about the child. As counselors, using this information can help us have far more effective insight into the student, which could help us have more informed conversations with the student's teachers and become better advocates for the students as well.

The psychological and educational testing results that might be discussed at the meeting can also be extremely helpful to a counselor. Understanding quantifiable levels of processing speed achievement or intelligence may help us set more realistic goals for our students. If, for example, the testing shows us that a student has an above average IQ but very slow processing speed, it becomes easier to understand why this otherwise extraordinary bright young person might not be answering questions in class. This understanding can lead to more effective advocacy on our part for our students. Of course, since students are so much more than their tests scores, these tests should never be used in isolation. In isolation from other assessment forms, an incomplete picture could be formed about the student. Used holistically, however, these tests can become very useful tools for counselors and other educators (Sattler, Dumont, & Coalson, 2016).

It is an unfortunate reality, however, that many counselors feel that with too many other responsibilities and far too much to do to fit into a day, an invitation to an IEP meeting may not be high on the list of important things to do, but we must remember that these opportunities for dialogue and collaboration are always in the best interest of our students.

Relationship with Child Study Team

For our students with learning disabilities to get the most comprehensive and appropriate services, child study team members and school counselors must be able to have an ongoing dialogue from the beginning about what is in the best interest of the student.

The relationship between the counselor and the child study team members needs to be collegial, respectful and based in an understanding of what each discipline is supposed to accomplish. Since each discipline has something unique and very specific to offer the student and the school, it would seem to make sense that counselors and members of the child study team should work hand in hand to provide their students with the very best of what they all have to offer.

An excellent place to start cultivating this relationship is at IEP meetings. In addition to gleaning all the useful information that is discussed at the IEP meeting in order to better help the student, we can also use these meetings to foster our relationship with the student's case manager and the members of the child study team in general. This partnership is a winning situation in every respect. For the student, a true partnership between their school counselor and the child study team creates a true multidisciplinary team with expertise in all aspects of their plan. For the child study team, this partnership results in the addition of another perspective from another qualified professional. For the counselor, this partnership results in learning more about the student's specific academic needs, which can then be used to advocate and work with the student more appropriately.

Unfortunately, this understanding and collaboration does not always occur. Research seems to indicate that there is still limited collaboration between school counselors and child study team members (Choi, Whitney, Korcuska, & Proctor, 2008). In addition, the lingering negative perception of the usefulness of counselors and confusion about what the role of the counselor actually is may also play a part in the lack of collaboration (Olanrewaju & Suleiman, 2019).

In short, the role of the school counselor is to help all students in academic, career and social/emotional development (ASCA, 2017). As counselors, we know that this translates into many different responsibilities during our day. We may be running groups on the same day that we are holding parent meetings, teaching classes or even proctoring tests. These varied responsibilities can create a lot of confusion over what our role really is. In contrast, the members of the child study team have clearly defined roles and goals. Typically, child study team members might be responsible for implementing IEPs, sharing that information with appropriate school personnel, conducting annual reviews, consulting with teachers, and managing the emotional and social needs of the classified student.

Ultimately, the goals of the child study team center on providing special education services and complying with the law. School counselors, on the other hand, although bound by the ethical standards of counseling, are not bound by the same legal obligations that are the crux of special education. Certainly the difference does not make any of these jobs any less difficult. Our jobs are equally stressful and equally fulfilling, but this contrast can play a part in the chasm that seems to exist between child study team members and school counselors. While our role as counselors may be misunderstood (Olanrewaju & Suleiman, 2019), the fact that the child study team's decisions have to be based on complying with the law is also something that gets misunderstood and because of this, it is sometimes difficult to find a neutral meeting ground. A functional system has to begin from a place of respect and understanding for what each discipline does and a desire to find the bridge between both worlds.

Identification

Another reason for cultivating mutual collaboration with the child study team is based on the fact that young students who have learning disabilities do not seem to be getting identified in a timely manner (Hallahan & Kauffman, 2006). Researchers have pointed to the fact that identification of students with learning disabilities before third grade has substantial positive effects on the academic progress of students with learning disabilities (Abreu-Ellis, Ellis, & Hayes, 2009; Goswami, 2008). Children who do not get identified before third grade tend to experience more academic challenges than children who are identified before third grade (Maughan, Rowe, Loeber, & Stouthamer-Loeber, 2003; NICHD, 2017). Although identification at any time is helpful (Shaywitz, 2003), the earlier the identification is done, the higher the chances of academic success for the student (Fuchs & Fuchs, 2006).

Although this early identification is considered to be key in helping students with learning disabilities (Abreu-Ellis et al., 2009; Goswami, 2008), it is not without its challenges. Early screening for learning disabilities can point out things such as low levels of phonemic awareness and letter knowledge that can be early predictors of potential learning disabilities (Muter & Snowling, 2009), but these predictors are not always trustworthy or easy to perceive (Hallahan & Kauffman, 2006). Since the range of normal development is quite vast and very young children do not typically engage in academic tasks, it is sometimes difficult to gauge what is a real learning disability and what might just be a mild delay (Hallahan & Kauffman, 2006). Another barrier to identification could lie in the fact that some young children mask their lack of decoding skills with memorization (Gray, 2008). For these children, while it may look as if they are decoding, they have actually just memorized the text and thus make it difficult to distinguish potential problems.

Unfortunately, as we can see, learning disabilities can be complex and difficult to identify early on (Hallahan & Kauffman, 2006), which makes accessing those important and early services and resources a very difficult task. In addition, another obstruction to identifying these students is the lack of training or support for teachers. Teachers, especially those in general education classes, have little information about learning disabilities. They are not typically trained in identifying possible learning disabilities. In fact, teachers in general education classrooms report that their preprofessional training programs did not require special coursework in special education (Blanton & Pugach, 2007; Cook et al., 2008). Many teachers report that in all of their preprofessional training, they have only had one special education course requirement and it was typically covered in very broad strokes (Blanton & Pugach, 2007). Researchers have actually suggested that only 5 out of every 100 students with dyslexia are ever identified or actually receive appropriate interventions (Dyslexia Research Institute, 2009).

Although the challenges involved in early identification may be great, it is still a first and necessary step toward providing the specific interventions, services and resources that children with learning disabilities require in order to succeed (Abreu-Ellis et al., 2009; Goswami, 2008).

So where does this leave us as counselors? Our knowledge of behavior, development and education places us in a position of responsibility with these children. The symptoms of learning disabilities do not end with having difficulty with academics. Externalizing behavior problems, lack of engagement and social/emotional issues go hand in hand with learning disabilities (Bennett, Brown, Boyle, Racine, & Offord, 2003; Maughan et al., 2003; Trzesniewski, Moffitt, Caspi, Taylor, & Maughan, 2006). What is really a learning disability may be coated with a mask of behavioral issues so thick that teachers may not even be able to look past them. These behaviors may actually preclude identification by teachers as they may not understand the underlying cycle of reading and learning problems, which may be at the root of the behavior (Tunmer & Greaney, 2010). The continued feelings of failure may create anxiety, depression, opposition and even school avoidance, but on the teacher's end, identification of a learning disability may be masked by the behavioral issues or disaffection (Tunmer & Greaney, 2010). Similarly, since there is a significant comorbidity between learning disabilities and attention deficit hyperactivity disorder (ADHD), the behaviors brought on by the ADHD (hyperactivity or inattention) may also work to preclude identification (Boada, Willcutt, & Pennington, 2012). Many of these children are also "frequent flyers" to the nurse's office. Their physical, somatic and frequent complaints may make them regular visitors to the school nurse and possible candidates for school avoidant behavior (DeBrew, 2014).

As elementary school counselors, these behaviors are not just signs that we need to work with these children emotionally. A wholistic evaluation of the crux of their issues needs to be done by us as well. Are they struggling academically? Are there problems in the home? Is there a history of learning disabilities in the family? Was the child born prematurely? These are all questions we need to ask in order to assess what to do next. Since learning disabilities do tend to run in families (Faraone et al., 1993) and are connected to prematurity (Cherkes-Julkowski, 1998) and are certainly connected to academic struggles, a child with all of these issues would certainly be a student who should be considered as a referral to the child study team for an evaluation.

References

Abreu-Ellis, C., Ellis, J., & Hayes, R. (2009). College preparedness and time of learning disability identification. *Journal of Developmental Education*, 32(3), 28.

ASCA. (2017). The essential role of elementary school counselors. Retrieved from https://www.schoolcounselor.org/asca/media/asca/Careers-Roles/WhyElem.pdf

Bennett, K. J., Brown, K. S., Boyle, M., Racine, Y., & Offord, D. (2003). Does low reading achievement at school entry cause conduct problems? *Social Science & Medicine*, 56(12), 2443–2448. https://doi.org/10.1016/S0277-9536(02)00247-2

Blanton, L. P., & Pugach, M. C. (2007). Collaborative programs in general and special teacher education. Council of Chief State School Officers, Washington, DC.

Boada, R., Willcutt, E. G., & Pennington, B. F. (2012). Understanding the comorbidity between dyslexia and attention-deficit/hyperactivity disorder. *Topics in Language Disorders*, 32(3), 264–284. http://dx.doi.org/10.1097/TLD.0b013e31826203ac

Cherkes-Julkowski, M. (1998). Learning disability, attention-deficit disorder, and language impairment as outcomes of prematurity: A longitudinal descriptive study. *Journal of Learning Disabilities*, 31(3), 294–306. https://doi.org/10.1177/002221949803100309

Choi, H., Whitney, Y., Korcuska, J. S., & Proctor, T. B. (2008). Consultation practices between school counselors and school psychologists: Implications for training and practice. *Journal of Applied School Psychology*, 24(2), 303–318. https://doi.org/10.1080/15377900802093348

Cook, C. R., Gresham, F. M., Kern, L., Barreras, R. B., Thornton, S., & Crews, S. D. (2008). Social skills training for secondary students with emotional and/or behavioral disorders: A review and analysis of the meta-analytic literature. *Journal of Emotional and Behavioral Disorders*, 16(3), 131–144. https://doi.org/10.1177/1063426608314541

DeBrew, J. K. (2014). An unlikely advocate: The role of the school nurse with children who have dyslexia. *NASN School Nurse*, 29(2), 60–62.

Dyslexia Research Institute. (2009). Mission statement. Retrieved from Dyslexia Research Institute website: http://www.dyslexia-add.org/index.html

Erford, B. T., & Erford, B. T. (2007). *Transforming the School Counseling Profession*. Columbus, GA: Pearson Merrill/Prentice Hall.

Faraone, S. V., Biederman, J., Lehman, B. K., Keenan, K., Norman, D., Seidman, L. J., … Chen, W. J. (1993). Evidence for the independent familial transmission of attention deficit hyperactivity disorder and learning disabilities: Results from a family genetic study. *The American Journal of Psychiatry*, 150(6), 891–895. http://dx.doi.org/10.1176/ajp.150.6.891

Fuchs, D., & Fuchs, L. S. (2006). Introduction to response to intervention: What, why, and how valid is it? *Reading Research Quarterly*, 41(1), 93–99. https://doi.org/10.1598/RRQ.41.1.4

Goswami, U. (2008). Reading, dyslexia and the brain. *Educational Research*, 50(2), 135–148. https://doi.org/10.1080/00131880802082625

Gray, E. S. (2008). Understanding dyslexia and its instructional implications: A case to support intense intervention. *Literacy Research and Instruction*, 47(2), 116–123. https://doi.org/10.1080/19388070701878790

Hallahan, D., & Kauffman, J. (2006). *Exceptional Learners: An Introduction to Special Education*. Boston, MA: Pearson.

Individuals with Disabilities Education Act (IDEA). (1997). Pub. L. No. 94–142, § 300.308.

Maughan, B., Rowe, R., Loeber, R., & Stouthamer-Loeber, M. (2003). Reading problems and depressed mood. *Journal of Abnormal Child Psychology*, 31(2), 219–229.

Muter, V., & Snowling, M. J. (2009). Children at familial risk of dyslexia: Practical implications from an at-risk study. *Child and Adolescent Mental Health*, 14(1), 37–41. https://doi.org/10.1111/j.1475-3588.2007.00480.x

NICHD. (2017). National Reading Panel. Retrieved from National Institute of Child Health and Human Development website: http://www.nichd.nih.gov/research/supported/Pages/nrp.aspx/

Olanrewaju, M. K., & Suleiman, Y. (2019). Perception assessment of guidance and counseling services among educational stakeholders in selected secondary schools in Oyo State, Nigeria. *Indonesian Journal of Educational Counseling*, 3(1), 31–42. https://doi.org/10.30653/001.201931.62

Sattler, M., Dumont, R., & Coalson, L. (2016). *Assessment of Children: WISC-V and WPPSI-IV*. San Diego: Jerome M. Sattler.

Shaywitz, S. (2003). *Overcoming Dyslexia: A New and Complete Science-Based Program for Reading Problems at any Level*. USA: Vintage Press.

Trzesniewski, K. H., Moffitt, T. E., Caspi, A., Taylor, A., & Maughan, B. (2006). Revisiting the association between reading achievement and antisocial behavior: New evidence of an environmental explanation from a twin study. *Child Development*, 77(1), 72–88. http://dx.doi.org/10.1111/j.1467–8624.2006.00857.x

Tunmer, W., & Greaney, K. (2010). Defining dyslexia. *Journal of Learning Disabilities*, 43(3), 229–243. http://dx.doi.org/10.1177/0022219409345009

8 Working with Teachers

In this part:

- Why work closely with teachers?
- How to best work collaboratively with teachers

Why Work Closely with Teachers?

Counselors who work with students with learning disabilities have a responsibility to their students to create a collaborative and positive relationship with teachers. This collaborative culture can lead to a much more successful outcome for all students but even more significantly for students with learning disabilities (Sink, 2008).

Studies have shown that there is a very powerful link between academic, social, self-management and motivational skills of students (Brigman & Campbell, 2003; Webb, Brigman, & Campbell, 2005). What this means is that if students with learning disabilities could work on their academic deficits with the same amount of focus and importance laid upon it as working on their social, self-management and motivational skills, then these students would have a much higher chance of finding academic success.

Collaboration between both general and special elementary school teachers and school counselors is pivotal in getting all of these areas addressed for students with learning disabilities. Working together as a team to achieve these goals leads to better outcomes for the students (Powers & Boes, 2013).

In addition to working with teachers collaboratively to get students' social–emotional needs met as well as their academics, it is important for counselors to be viewed as a respected and valued part of the team for the students (Mayes, Dollahide, & Young, 2018). When a counselor sees a need to advocate for a student's needs, a teacher who views the counselor as a peer as opposed to as an adversary would be more likely to work with the counselor in a way that would benefit the student.

How to Best Work Collaboratively with Teachers

Students do best when the approach to their education, including their social–emotional education, is seamless (Goddard, Goddard, & Tschannen-Moran, 2007). In this way, there are several models that work best when trying to create a collaborative atmosphere between counselors and teachers.

There are many ways that counselors can help create a collaborative environment with teachers. Although each method is an independent method, all of these methods should work together to create the best possible climate for collaboration and, ultimately, for the well-being of the students (Hallam, Smith, Hite, Hite, & Wilcox, 2015).

One way to create a collaborative environment is to involve the teacher as much as possible (Hallam et al., 2015). Elementary school teachers are the main adult in the school for small children, and many elementary school teachers take great pride in their relationships with their students. Since confidentiality is at the core of the counseling profession, we have to take great care in not divulging information to anyone who has not been given that privilege. Approaching this confidentiality from the perspective of respect for all parties involved gives equal acknowledgment of the importance of the confidential information as well as the importance of the role of the teacher in the life of the student. Telling a teacher that you cannot share information with them must be done in a way that does not alienate the teacher, while at the same time allowing for the confidential information to remain confidential. The last thing we want to do is alienate the person who can work with us in a positive way to help this child the most.

As a collaborator with teachers, one method that is helpful is for the counselor to play a consultant role (Warren & Robinson, 2015). Of course, for the teacher to come to the counselor in this capacity, trust must be established from the beginning. The counselor must meet the teacher "where they are." If a teacher is completely ingrained in social–emotional learning and is open and ready to learn about learning disabilities, then there is no problem. Your willing audience is right there. On the other hand, when a teacher feels the strain of having to cover too much material and you show up at their door with pamphlets and lesson plans about something they may not have so much faith in to begin with, you may have to tread a little more lightly and work with them more slowly. Although the end result is the best interest of the student, the path to getting there is frequently with the help of their teacher.

General education teachers who have students with learning disabilities in their classrooms may not have appropriate information for managing these students. Since most general education teachers do not normally receive very much preservice training for learning disabilities (Mackey & Greenfield, 2018), this is not a surprise. It might be helpful to work with these teachers and give them guidelines for helping students with learning disabilities.

HOW TO HELP A STUDENT WITH DYSLEXIA

In this part:

- Typical hallmarks of dyslexia
- Tip sheet for teachers: Dyslexia

Typical Hallmarks of Dyslexia

Understand that a student with dyslexia may:

- Have difficulty rhyming
- Have difficulty articulating well
- Have difficulty counting syllables
- Be avoidant of academic work (they may frequently ask to go to the nurse, the bathroom or to sharpen their pencils)
- Communicate their knowledge better in oral form
- Seem more tired than the other students
- Have some behavioral issues
- Have difficulty with charts and graphs
- Believe that they are stupid
- Have days when they know the material and then days when they don't
- Struggle with new words or forget words
- Have difficulty concentrating
- Have difficulty understanding idioms
- Have difficulty following sequential directions
- Hand in messy papers
- Not complete homework
- Confuse similar looking letters or reverse letters (but this is not the hallmark of dyslexia)
- Have unusual pronunciation of words
- Have unusual pencil grip
- Not produce work that seems appropriate to their ability
- Miss words when reading out loud
- Have difficulty with supporting an argument or getting to the point
- Not recognize words that should be familiar
- Have low self-esteem
- Have difficulty remembering the order of things, such as the days of the week or months of the year
- Have difficulty learning to tell time, or remembering dates, phone numbers and birthdays
- Not know the difference between right and left
- Be withdrawn or have externalizing behavior issues
- Have difficulty remembering the names of people and/or places
- Struggle with learning foreign languages (British Dyslexia Association, 2017; Goswami, 2008; International Dyslexia Organization, 2015; Lyon, 1995; NICHD, 2017; Shaywitz, 2003)

Please note that although many people experience challenges, a student with dyslexia may exhibit several of these challenges simultaneously.

Tip Sheet for Teachers: Dyslexia

- Give directions clearly and one direction at a time
- Place value on tenacity and effort as opposed to grades
- Give positive attention
- Monitor long-term assignments
- Allow alternate assessment methods
- Give study guides if appropriate (older grades)
- Teach mnemonics
- Help student create flash cards
- Minimize distractions
- Break up big projects
- Provide opportunities for success
- Allow use of audio books
- Allow dictation of written responses
- Incorporate social–emotional learning into the day-to-day teaching (British Dyslexia Association, 2017; Goswami, 2008; International Dyslexia Organization, 2015; Lyon, 1995; NICHD, 2017; Shaywitz, 2003)

Please note that although many people experience challenges, a student with dyslexia may exhibit several of these challenges simultaneously.

HOW TO HELP A STUDENT WITH DYSCALCULIA

In this part:

- Typical hallmarks of dyscalculia
- Tip sheet for teachers: Dyscalculia

Typical Hallmarks of Dyscalculia

Understand that a student with dyscalculia may:

- Have difficulty with mathematical word problems
- Have difficulty understanding money concepts or making change
- Be challenged by the concepts of positive and negative value, number lines, place value, carrying and borrowing
- Have difficulty lining up numbers on a page for calculation
- Have challenges with sequencing information or events
- Have difficulty with multistep math problems
- Have difficulty recognizing patterns

- Have difficulty attaching a number to the quantity it represents
- May lose track of time
- May have externalizing behaviors, anxiety or depression
- Have difficulty with time-related concepts, such as days, weeks or months (Kuhn, 2015; Shalev, 2001)

Tip Sheet for Teachers: Dyscalculia

- Allow extra time for tests
- Perform frequent (but not obvious) checks for understanding
- Break down multistep problems into clearly stated simple steps
- Allow student to narrate math problems
- Allow student to use graph paper for lining up numbers and columns
- Provide sample problems
- Allow use of whiteboards
- Give extra instruction on basic math facts
- Create connections to math from prior experiences
- Teach and allow use of calculator
- Review material frequently
- Help student find patterns within the work
- Explain and correct errors quickly
- Place value on student growth over grades
- Praise effort over outcome
- Allow timers to help student keep track of time
- Acknowledge possible embarrassment over not knowing math facts
- Allow student to answer questions when their hands are raised rather than calling on them
- Establish signals for letting the teacher know that the student feels confident in answering questions
- Address the anxiety
- Help the student realize that their disability does not define their intelligence
- Help the student realize that they are more than their disability
- Never say "this is easy"
- Teach breathing exercises to use before tests and assessments (Haberstroh & Schulte-Körne, 2019; Kucian & von Aster, 2015)

HOW TO HELP A STUDENT WITH DYSGRAPHIA

In this part:

- Typical hallmarks of dysgraphia
- Tip sheet for teachers: Dysgraphia

Typical Hallmarks of Dysgraphia

Understand that a student with dysgraphia may:

- Have an awkward pencil grip
- Have illegible printing and cursive
- May use print and cursive together, have inconsistent spacing, interchange upper and lowercase letters, or use irregular-sized or shaped letters
- Omit words or letters
- Have difficulty copying or writing in a timely manner
- Have unusual spatial planning on paper
- Complain of hand pain or tiredness
- Have difficulty thinking and writing simultaneously
- Have difficulty speaking words aloud while writing
- Exhibit avoidant behavior toward writing tasks
- Exhibit poor organization of thoughts in written form
- Have poor syntax or grammar
- Have good verbal ideas but difficulty with executing ideas in writing
- Have unusual spelling errors
- Exhibit very slow or very fast writing
- Exhibit frustration and stress when tasked with writing (Mayes, Breaux, Calhoun, & Frye, 2017)

Tip Sheet for Teachers: Dysgraphia

- Accommodate with
  - Larger pens or pencils
  - Raised lines on paper
  - Audio recorders
  - Speech-to-text programs
  - Compensatory skills (such as keyboarding)
- Modify with
  - Breaking down larger written assignments
  - Focusing on content
  - Alternative formats for written assignments
  - Reducing writing length or complexity
- Remediate with
  - Motor tasks (clay and putty, tracing letters)
  - Hand exercises
  - Good posture and pencil grip
  - Specific letter writing instruction
- Provide specific and pointed instruction in letter formation
- Teach the use of graphic organizers
- Teach proofreading

- Allow extra time on tests
- Allow graph paper for math
- Remove neatness as part of the grade (Chung & Patel, 2015)

HOW TO HELP A STUDENT WITH PROCESSING DISORDERS (VISUAL AND AUDITORY)

In this part:

- Typical hallmarks of processing disorders (visual and auditory)
- Tip sheet for teachers: Processing disorders (visual and auditory)

Typical Hallmarks of Processing Disorders (Visual and Auditory)

Understand that a student with visual processing disorder may:

- Have difficulty with perceiving objects in front of or behind other objects
- Have difficulty learning and understanding the difference between left and right, or up and down
- Have challenges with discriminating color, form, shape, pattern, size and position
- Have difficulty reading charts and graphs
- Have difficulty recognizing common objects
- Have inconsistent recognition of numbers and letters
- Display challenges understanding the difference between a whole and its parts
- Display challenges with fine and gross motor skills
- Seem distracted when presented with too much visual information
- Display difficulty copying from the board
- Reverse numbers, letters and words
- Have difficulty remembering phone numbers
- Frequently complain that their eyes hurt
- Skip words or lines when reading
- Omit steps and confuse formulas in math problems
- Not notice new or changed signs in a familiar environment (Arky, 2018; National Center for Learning Disabilities, 2005)

Understand that a student with auditory processing disorder may:

- Have difficulty in recognizing phonemes
- Have difficulty following verbal instructions
- Have auditory sequencing issues (i.e., "tevelision" instead of "television")
- Pronounce obviously different words similarly

- Be unable to tease out important sounds or follow conversations in a noisy environment
- Have difficulty with reading and spelling
- Have oral math issues
- Have poor musical ability
- Display challenges with learning rhymes or songs
- Not speak clearly
- Have social skills issues
- Have comorbidity with dyslexia, ADHD and other related conditions (Johnson, 2018)

Tip Sheet for Teachers: Processing Disorders (Visual and Auditory)

Auditory

- Repeat information frequently and clearly
- Allow the student a preview of information prior to learning it in class
- Allow the student to sit closest to the learning
- Limit distractions
- Help the student by chunking information
- Provide visual cues for responses
- Give clear and concrete directions
- Allow extra time for processing time – count to ten slowly before expecting a response
- Provide frequent yet unobtrusive checks for understanding
- Teach note-taking skills as appropriate

Visual

- Chunk assignments into smaller steps
- Provide writing paper with dark or raised lines
- Make sure that worksheets that are visually "clean" and not overly distracting
- Allow for alternative methods of displaying understanding
- Limiting copying from board

HOW TO HELP A STUDENT WITH NONVERBAL LEARNING DISORDER

In this part:

- Typical hallmarks of nonverbal learning disorder
- Tip sheet for teachers: Nonverbal learning disorder

Typical Hallmarks of Nonverbal Learning Disorder

Understand that a student with nonverbal learning disorder may:

- Have difficulty recognizing nonverbal cues
- Display poor reading comprehension despite large vocabulary
- Have shown very early and precocious language acquisition and advanced verbal skills
- Have gross and fine motor skills issues
- Appear clumsy and have difficulty with fine motor skills, such as using scissors
- Ask frequent and repetitive questions
- Display difficulty understanding idioms or spatial information
- Be very literal and have challenges understanding sarcasm
- Show difficulty with handling changes in life or routine
- Not understand nonverbal cues and may seem overly trusting
- Have trouble following multistep directions
- Have difficulty understanding generalizations
- Have difficulties in math computation, science, writing and reading comprehension (Franz, 2000)

Tip Sheet for Teachers: Nonverbal Learning Disorder

- Provide explicit and direct instruction
- Help student create connections to new learning from previous learning
- Reduce visually distracting information on worksheets
- Provide clear, concise and immediate verbal feedback
- Minimize distractions
- Provide frequent checks for understanding
- Teach compensatory skills (such as keyboarding) while still remediating
- Provide examples for problem-solving questions
- Teach a variety of problem-solving skills
- Teach how to use graphic organizers
- Allow speech-to-text programs for alternate methods of response
- Allow narration of math problems
- Provide graph paper for math problems

HOW TO HELP A STUDENT WITH ADHD

In this part:

- Typical hallmarks of ADHD
- Tip sheet for teachers: ADHD

Typical Hallmarks of ADHD

Understand that a student with ADHD may:

General

- Have difficulty with following instructions
- Have challenges with organization
- Leave projects unfinished
- Have difficulty paying attention to details
- Have poor academic performance
- Have difficulty with relationships
- Display social issues
- Have disciplinary issues (Noorbala & Akhondzadeh, 2006)

Inattentive

- Miss details
- Struggle with maintaining attention
- Be easily sidetracked by other projects
- Frequently not complete projects
- Have difficulty with sequencing
- Have poor time management
- Hand in messy classwork or homework
- Have a very messy room, locker and backpack
- Display challenges with meeting deadlines or being on time
- Avoid tasks that require sustained attention
- Lose unexpected things (coats in winter, glasses, etc.)
- Be easily distracted by everything
- Forget appointments
- Suffer from anxiety and/or depression (Noorbala & Akhondzadeh, 2006)

Hyperactivity

- Frequently squirm and fidget in seat at school
- Leave seat unexpectedly
- Display frequent restlessness
- Have difficulty playing quietly
- Talk constantly
- Shout out answers
- Interrupt people frequently
- Have difficulty taking turns
- Lack inhibition
- Have impulsive behavior (Noorbala & Akhondzadeh, 2006)

Tip Sheet for Teachers: ADHD

- Provide consistent and clear rules
- Provide consistent daily routines
- Reduce distractions for test taking, homework or classwork
- Provide direct instruction in organizational methods
- Provide direct monitoring of organization early on in order to establish routines
- Provide notice prior to changes in activity or for transitions
- Provide extended time
- Shorten assignments (at first) to provide opportunities for success and to encourage engagement
- Help student create color-coded notebooks
- Provide class notes as appropriate
- Praise frequently and provide positive reinforcement
- Acknowledge frustrations
- Set up system of nonverbal signals to encourage refocusing (Post-it note on desk, tapping on desk, etc.)
- Provide a clearly written schedule
- Create specific places to store frequently used items (pencils in pencil box, books in cubby, etc.)
- Help student set up notebook organizers and planners
- Provide direct instruction in the use of calendars, lists and reminder notes
- Break down large tasks

HOW TO HELP A STUDENT WITH DYSPRAXIA

In this part:

- Typical hallmarks of dyspraxia
- Tip sheet for teachers: Dyspraxia

Typical Hallmarks of Dyspraxia

Understand that a student with dyspraxia may:

- Have poor balance or clumsy movements
- Have difficulty with fine and gross motor skills
- Have challenges with coordinating both sides of the body simultaneously
- Have hand–eye coordination challenges
- Find organizing themselves challenging and difficult
- Be sensitive to touch

- Have poor handwriting
- Have spelling and reading problems
- Be upset by loud or constant noises
- Have social and emotional difficulties
- Be challenged by time management
- Have difficulty with memory
- Have processing issues
- Have speech articulation difficulties
- Display sensory issues related to clothing
- Have poor spatial awareness and difficulty judging speed or distance
- Have poor stamina
- Have difficulty adapting to new situations
- Be very literal
- Be immature
- Have difficulty remembering or following instructions
- Have extreme emotions
- Lack understanding of potential danger (Learning Disabilities Association, 2018)

Tip Sheet for Teachers: Dyspraxia

- Accept them for who they are
- Reassure them that they are wonderful just as they are
- Give specific and honest praise on both effort and performance
- Set reasonable and realistic goals based on student's actual abilities
- Provide early instruction in keyboarding
- Give specific and constructive responses to work
- Provide extra time to compensate for slow processing of information
- Break new tasks and information into smaller chunks
- Allow for time to practice
- Provide instruction of specific skills with an eye toward generalizing
- Provide step-by-step checklists for learning
- State directions clearly and simply
- Minimize visual distractions
- Teach using multiple modalities

HOW TO HELP A STUDENT WITH EXECUTIVE FUNCTION DISORDER

In this part:

- Typical hallmarks of executive function disorder
- Tip sheet for teachers: Executive function disorder

Typical Hallmarks of Executive Function Disorder

Understand that a student with executive function disorder may:

- Have difficulty making plans
- Display difficulty keeping track of time
- Have difficulty keeping track of more than one thing at a time
- Show an inability to finish work on time
- Have difficulty planning long-range projects
- Have difficulty discussing details sequentially
- Have difficulty with memorizing and retrieval
- Be challenged by starting tasks (Semrud-Clikeman, Pliszka, & Liotti, 2008)

Tip Sheet for Teachers: Executive Function Disorder

- Provide step-by-step instructions
- Create clear routines
- Provide student with prior access to contents of new lesson
- Provide frequent checks for understanding
- Give clear, concise and simple directions
- Help student create to-do lists or checklists
- Help student chunk information into smaller bits
- Allow speech-to-text software or verbal responses
- Break large goals into smaller parts
- Allow planned breaks
- Use timers for clear delineation of activities
- Provide direct instruction in the use of organizational materials
- Allow for rewards for positive behavior
- Teach mnemonic devices and skills

HOW TO HELP A STUDENT WITH MEMORY ISSUES

In this part:

- Typical hallmarks of working memory issues
- Tip sheet for teachers: Working memory issues
- Typical hallmarks of short-term memory issues
- Tip sheet for teachers: Short-term memory issues

Typical Hallmarks of Working Memory Issues

Understand that a student with working memory issues may:

- Have a quiet affect in large groups
- Suffer from inattention and distraction

- Have issues with executive function
- Display difficulty with planning
- Have problem-solving difficulties
- Have issues with sustaining attention
- Have trouble with following through on directions even if the directions are understood
- Have difficulty with multiple-step math calculations
- Have word problem difficulties
- Have reading comprehension issues
- Have writing composition difficulties
- Have difficulty with higher-order thinking tasks (Holmes, Gathercole, & Dunning, 2010; Kail & Hall, 2001)

Tip Sheet for Teachers: Working Memory Issues

- Teach compensatory strategies
- Give student written sequential steps for problem solving
- Provide written schedules
- Connect new ideas to older and more familiar ones
- Chunk information into smaller segments
- Provide extra time for review
- Provide extra academic support for new learning tasks
- Model steps in multistep problems
- Check for understanding frequently and unobtrusively

Typical Hallmarks of Short-Term Memory Issues

Understand that a student with short-term memory issues may:

- Have difficulties in speech and language
- Have difficulties with multistep math problems
- Have difficulty remembering what was just heard (Alexander, 2004)

Tip Sheet for Teachers: Short-Term Memory Issues

- Provide lists or checklists
- Help student organize or create calendars
- Teach student how to use mnemonic devices
- Allow student to use open-note or open-book exams
- Use a multisensory teaching approach
- Allow use of computers
- Maintain routines as much as possible
- Use repetition as a teaching tool

References

Alexander, T. (2004). Memory/Recall Difficulties. Retrieved from Strategies for Creating Inclusive Programmes of Study website: https://scips.worc.ac.uk/challenges/memory/

Arky, B. (2018). Understanding Visual Processing Issues. Retrieved from https://www.understood.org/en/learning-attention-issues/child-learning-disabilities/visual-processing-issues/understanding-visual-processing-issues

Brigman, G., & Campbell, C. (2003). Helping students improve academic achievement and school success behavior. *Professional School Counseling*, 7(2), 91–98.

British Dyslexia Association. (2017). Screening and Assessment. *British Dyslexia Association*, 8(8). Retrieved from http://www.bdadyslexia.org.uk/educator/screening-and-assessment

Chung, P., & Patel, D. R. (2015). Dysgraphia. *International Journal of Child and Adolescent Health*, 8(1), 27.

Franz, C. (2000). Diagnosis and Management of Nonverbal Learning Disorders. Paper presented at the *Annual Convention of the National Association of School Psychologists*, New Orleans, LA. Retrieved from https://eric.ed.gov

Goddard, Y. L., Goddard, R. D., & Tschannen-Moran, M. (2007). A theoretical and empirical investigation of teacher collaboration for school improvement and student achievement in public elementary schools. *Teachers College Record*, 109(4), 877–896.

Goswami, U. (2008). Reading, dyslexia and the brain. *Educational Research*, 50(2), 135–148. https://doi.org/10.1080/00131880802082625

Haberstroh, S., & Schulte-Körne, G. (2019). The diagnosis and treatment of dyscalculia. *Deutsches Ärzteblatt International*, 116(7), 107. https://doi.org/10.3238/arztebl.2019.0107

Hallam, P. R., Smith, H. R., Hite, J. M., Hite, S. J., & Wilcox, B. R. (2015). Trust and collaboration in PLC teams: Teacher relationships, principal support, and collaborative benefits. *NASSP Bulletin*, 99(3), 193–216. https://doi.org/10.1177/0192636515602330

Holmes, J., Gathercole, S. E., & Dunning, D. L. (2010). Poor working memory: Impact and interventions. *Advances in Child Development and Behavior*, 39, 1–43.

International Dyslexia Organization. (2015). International Dyslexia Organization Fact Sheet. Retrieved from http://eida.org/fact-sheets/

Johnson, K. (2018). Understanding Auditory Processing Disorder. Retrieved from Understood website: https://www.understood.org/en/learning-attention-issues/child-learning-disabilities/auditory-processing-disorder/understanding-auditory-processing-disorder

Kail, R., & Hall, L. (2001). Distinguishing short-term memory from working memory. *Memory and Cognition*, 29(1), 1–9.

Kucian, K., & von Aster, M. (2015). Developmental dyscalculia. *European Journal of Pediatrics*, 174(1), 1–13.

Kuhn, J.-T. (2015). Developmental dyscalculia. *Zeitschrift Für Psychologie*, 223(2), 69–82. https://doi.org/10.1027/2151-2604/a000205

Learning Disabilities Association. (2018). Dyspraxia. Retrieved from Learning Disabilities Association website: https://ldaamerica.org/types-of-learning-disabilities/dyspraxia/

Lyon, G. R. (1995). Toward a definition of dyslexia. *Annals of Dyslexia*, 45(1), 1–27. https://doi.org/10.1007/BF02648210

Mackey, M., & Greenfield, R. (2018). Pre-service teachers' perceptions of learning disabilities: Examining effectiveness of special education coursework. Retrieved from The Qualitative Report Conference website: https://nsuworks. nova.edu/tqrc/ninth/day1/24/

Mayes, R. D., Dollahide, C. T., & Young, A. (2018). School counselors as leaders in school turnaround. *Journal of Organizational and Educational Leadership*, 4(1), 1–24.

Mayes, S. D., Breaux, R. P., Calhoun, S. L., & Frye, S. S. (2017). High prevalence of dysgraphia in elementary through high school students with ADHD and autism. *Journal of Attention Disorders*, 23(8), 787–796. https://doi. org/10.1177/1087054717720721

National Center for Learning Disabilities. (2008). Executive Function Fact Sheet. Retrieved from LD Online: http://www.ldonline.org/article/24880/

NICHD. (2017). National Reading Panel. Retrieved from National Institute of Child Health and Human Development website: http://www.nichd.nih.gov/ research/supported/Pages/nrp.aspx/

Noorbala, A.-A., & Akhondzadeh, S. (2006). Attention-deficit/hyperactivity disorder: Etiology and pharmacotherapy. *Arch Iran Med*, 9(4), 374–80.

Powers, P., & Boes, S. R. (2013). Steps toward understanding: Teacher perceptions of the school counselor role. *Georgia School Counselors Association Journal*, 20(1), n1.

Semrud-Clikeman, M., Pliszka, S. R., & Liotti, M. (2008). Executive functioning in children with attention-deficit/hyperactivity disorder: Combined type with and without a stimulant medication history. *Neuropsychology (Journal)*, 22(3), 329–340. https://doi.org/10.1037/0894-4105.22.3.329

Shalev, R. (2001). Developmental dyscalculia. *Journal of Child Neurology*, 19(10), 765–771. https://doi.org/10.1177/08830738040190100601

Shaywitz, S. (2003). *Overcoming Dyslexia: A New and Complete Science-Based Program for Reading Problems at Any Level*. USA: Vintage Press.

Sink, C. A. (2008). Elementary school counselors and teachers: Collaborators for higher student achievement. *The Elementary School Journal*, 108(5), 445–458. https://doi.org/10.1086/589473

Warren, J. M., & Robinson, G. (2015). Addressing barriers to effective RTI through school counselor consultation: A social justice approach. *Electronic Journal for Inclusive Education*, 3(4), 3.

Webb, L. D., Brigman, G. A., & Campbell, C. (2005). Linking school counselors and student success: A replication of the Student Success Skills approach targeting the academic and social competence of students. *Professional School Counseling*, 8(5), 407–413.

9 Working with Parents

In this part:

- Why is it important?
- How can we involve parents?

Why Is It Important?

When elementary school counselors work closely with parents, wonderful things happen. Research has shown that parental involvement is a significant factor in student achievement (Trusty, Mellin, & Herbert, 2008).

For parents of students with special needs, this involvement becomes even more important. In general, the research suggests that parents of students with special needs tend to be less involved to begin with (Fishman & Nickerson, 2015). Given this fact, involving these parents becomes even more important and increases the likelihood the young students with learning disabilities will become successful.

How Can We Involve Parents?

One of the best ways we can involve parents in working in the best interest of their children with learning disabilities is to involve them as partners and to empower them with the knowledge that will help them advocate best for their children. Since parents with special needs tend to be less involved in the education of their children to begin with (Fishman & Nickerson, 2015), the information they may need to best help their children may not have been available to them. We can provide parents with individual or group parent meetings where we can teach important and relevant aspects about parenting students with learning disabilities. Some of the most important information that could be related to these parents could be the following:

1. Understanding the relationship between parent involvement and student success (Walker, Shenker, & Hoover-Dempsey, 2010). Researchers have shown a positive correlation between parent

involvement and student success. As counselors, we can be the school leaders who can encourage this involvement and help to create positive benefits for all children, not just students with learning disabilities. For students with learning disabilities, this involvement becomes even more important. If parental involvement can make a positive impact on students who do not display learning disabilities, then the impact that parental involvement can make with students who do have learning disabilities is even more significant. When we look at the research that makes a connection between students with learning disabilities and lack of success in later school it becomes clear that creating a culture of parental involvement, especially for these students, can do nothing but help.

2. Appropriate parenting interventions (Tarver, Daley, & Sayal, 2015). Parenting can be difficult enough with students without learning disabilities, but when a parent has a child, or even several children, with learning disabilities, it becomes even more challenging. A child with a learning disability without externalizing behaviors in school may come home frustrated, angry and exhausted. This child may display a shortened temper, an inability to deal with even the slightest adversity and complete lack of desire to do any kind of homework. A child with a learning disability with externalizing behaviors in school can become frustrating to deal with at home as well.

3. An understanding of what learning disabilities are and how they manifest (Gold & Richmond, 1979). Parents may not innately understand the academic struggles that their children are having due to their learning disabilities. These struggles may be interpreted as laziness, frustration or plain recalcitrance. Giving parents the opportunity to begin to learn all of the surprising ways that learning disabilities can manifest changes the whole trajectory of parenting.

4. Understanding how to be your child's advocate (Gold & Richmond, 1979). It is not always easy to be an appropriate advocate for a child with a learning disability. For parents who are watching their children struggle, it is sometimes easier to blame the environment, the teacher or the school before looking at the behavior of their own child. Becoming an effective advocate for a child with a learning disability involves being able to tease out where the problem actually lies. Although parents should not always think that every single thing that their child does is wrong, thinking that every single thing that their child does is perfect is also not helpful.

5. How and why to help your children maintain a positive attitude (Gold & Richmond, 1979). Parents of children with learning disabilities should be given an understanding of the importance of a positive attitude. Students who continued to feel good about themselves as learners, with or without learning disabilities, tend to stay engaged in school and tend to find academic success even later on. It is important

for parents to be the appropriate cheerleaders for their children on an ongoing basis. The challenge with this role for parents of children with learning disabilities is that there is a fine line between being the cheerleader and negating the frustrations and challenges of their child's learning disability. It is reasonable to explain to parents that it is just as appropriate to acknowledge their child's frustration while still pushing them forward in a positive and encouraging manner. Similarly, it is also important to make sure that parents understand that positive praise that is unwarranted can actually have a negative impact. Parents can be taught to give specific praise. For example, a student who has just failed a math test should not be praised and told that they are good at math. This unwarranted praise will confuse them and make them stop trusting the praise that parents give them. Instead, they can be told that their effort in studying for the test was wonderful and that because they have a learning disability sometimes it makes doing well on tests difficult but it doesn't mean but they are not intelligent and engaged students. In this instance, parents can also be taught to say something like, "This only teaches us that you might still need help learning this material. We can talk to your teacher and review more and then we can see how you do then."

References

Fishman, C. E., & Nickerson, A. B. (2015). Motivations for involvement: A preliminary investigation of parents of students with disabilities. *Journal of Child and Family Studies*, 24(2), 523–535.

Gold, P., & Richmond, L. J. (1979). Counseling parents of learning disabled children. *Elementary School Guidance & Counseling*, 14(1), 16–21. Retrieved from JSTOR.

Tarver, J., Daley, D., & Sayal, K. (2015). Beyond symptom control for attention-deficit hyperactivity disorder (ADHD): What can parents do to improve outcomes? *Child: Care, Health and Development*, 41(1), 1–14. https://doi.org/10.1111/cch.12159

Trusty, J., Mellin, E. A., & Herbert, J. T. (2008). Closing achievement gaps: Roles and tasks of elementary school counselors. *The Elementary School Journal*, 108(5), 407–421. https://doi.org/10.1086/589470

Walker, J. M., Shenker, S. S., & Hoover-Dempsey, K. V. (2010). Why do parents become involved in their children's education? Implications for school counselors. *Professional School Counseling*, 14(1), 27–41.

10 The Program

In this part:

- Developing the program
- Creating buy-in
- Finding group members
- General instructions for the group

Developing the Program

The program presented in this book is meant to be used by school counselors in a school or a clinical setting with kindergarten through fifth-grade students. The groups should be broken up into two groups: one group should be kindergarten to grade three while the other should be grade four to grade five. While the provided lessons break the groups up at these grade levels, the counselor should feel free to mix and match according to their own students' maturity levels and abilities. Membership in the group is based on the student having an individualized education plan (IEP), a 504 plan, or a suspected learning disability or learning challenge. The group is meant to be voluntary (at this age level it would be primarily based on parental desire for their child to attend) and should have anywhere from four to ten members.

Creating Buy-In

Successful programs must be built with a bigger picture in mind. In a school system, the system itself has a voice in dictating how and why programs exist or don't. Getting buy-in from all parties is therefore important and necessary in order to ensure the success of the program. Administrators, supervisors, teachers, parents and students should all have a sense of the importance and usefulness of the program in order for it to become a viable service. In order for any program to be seen as useful by the community, the need for its existence has to be explained and accepted. Many programs develop based on the findings of needs assessments. The needs assessments survey the needs of the community and then programs are created in order to serve these needs. For this program, however, the need does not become blatantly obvious until after the students have left elementary school. These students may have teachers who work with them so closely that they will not "fail" their elementary program, but once they get to middle school, high school and beyond, they may not be able to succeed without that intense help. For this reason, it is important to have all stakeholders understand that the need for this program is more global in scale. The need for helping these children lies in all of the empirical evidence that suggests that students with learning disabilities are not being prepared to succeed in college. We can get these students to college but once they get there, they are almost 20% more likely to drop out than are their peers without learning disabilities (Cortiella & Horowitz, 2014). The earlier the intervention for these students, the more likely that they will be successful later on (Cortiella & Horowitz, 2014). In terms of the school counselor's role, even though college success may not seem to have much to do with the elementary school counselor's role, a student's self-perception as a learner begins as soon as that student walks into a school. This self-perception is at the crux of a student's ability to learn. If a student believes in themselves as a learner and is given all of the tools that have been shown to create academic success for students with learning disabilities, such as understanding themselves as learners, understanding their strengths and challenges and learning to advocate for themselves (among other things!), then these students have a higher chance at finding academic success. The research indicates that students in elementary school who present with social skills deficits, inattention and learning issues are not finding long-term academic success (Rabiner, Godwin, & Dodge, 2016). These students have a higher likelihood of becoming incarcerated, suffering from depression, being unemployed, dropping out of high school and college, or just not attending college at all (Cortiella & Horowitz, 2014; Fitzpatrick, Archambault, Janosz, & Pagani, 2015; Shapiro et al., 2017). This is the information that will be necessary for getting all stakeholders to buy into the necessity for the program.

For teachers, creating buy-in is also very important. Few teachers want their students out of their class even more than they get pulled out already. Teachers then also need to be a part of the discussion. Involving them by explaining the program or getting input about best times for scheduling is helpful. In general, being respectful of teachers and their curricular needs is just good practice no matter what the reason.

Approaching other stakeholders such as administrators is also a necessary part of the creation of the program. A well-designed and thoughtful plan partnered with appropriate justification is key to getting buy-in. You will need the following information:

- Justification for the group (described earlier)
- An overview of the program itself
- An idea of how many participants there will be
- An idea of the timeframe
- Weekly topics
- A plan for finding members
- A plan for notifying parents
- A plan for parental permission if needed
- A plan for establishing meeting times
- A plan for the structure of the group

Finding Group Members

In general, any student who already has an IEP or a 504 might be eligible for the group. As counselors, we may be able to have access to IEPs or 504s. If this information is available, any student with a classification of "Specific Learning Disability" or possibly "Other Health Impaired" might be eligible. More specifically, if a student (who is not profoundly impaired) is displaying academic difficulties (including attentional and behavioral difficulties as well as specific learning lags), then they would be eligible for the group whether or not they have been classified. Speaking to teachers and asking for input is an excellent way to identify which students might have these needs.

At this point, it is time to approach the parents. An initial email followed by a personal phone call can start the ball rolling. Having teachers or child study team members reach out to the parents (who may not know or trust the counselor) is also very helpful. A follow-up email can explain the group in more detail and can contain a schedule. Consent forms, if needed, can be sent at this time.

General Instructions for the Group

Lessons in this program are not meant to be followed to the letter but rather are meant to be used as a starting point for discussion. A counselor's level of comfort and experience can determine what the needs are at the time for each particular group. In general, the overarching concept are what needs to be taught. The framework presented here is a guide for teaching the concepts but in no way is this the only way to get this done. What is important is to always make certain that the research-based topics that are the crux of the lessons are always touched upon during the weeks of the group.

GOAL SETTING LESSON PLAN

Kindergarten to Third Grade

Materials:

> Whiteboard, chart paper or board
> Marker or chalk
> Handout 1.1 – Go for the Goal!
> Handout 1.2 – Goal Chart for Classrooms (if needed)

Say the following:

- Today we will be discussing goal setting.
- Before we talk more about what goal setting is, I want to tell you a secret about myself.

    I want to learn how to fly in the air like a bird! I don't want to be in a plane; I just want to spread my arms out and fly, just like birds do.

- Is it possible for me to learn to fly in the air just like a bird?

(*Allow for responses.*)

- Why is it not possible?

(*Allow for responses.*)

- You are right! It is not possible because I am *not* a bird and I don't have wings like a bird. If my secret wish is to learn how to fly, then my secret wish is not going to happen.
- But what if my secret wish is to learn how to read better? Can that happen?

(*Allow for responses.*)

- Yes! Of course I can learn how to read better. That is something that is possible *and* it is something that I want to get good or better at. Goals must be possible and have to be something you want to get good or better at.
- My wish to fly like a bird is more like a dream, but my wish to learn to read better is a goal.
- What is a big difference between goals and dreams?

(*Allow for responses.*)

- Yes! Dreams can be about anything. You can dream that you want to be a fish in the ocean. You can dream that you want to be a dinosaur, but goals must be something that is possible and be something that you can get good or better at.
- You will all have to help me with this next part. I'm going to tell you something that I want to achieve, and you tell me whether it is a dream or a goal. Ready?

- I want to be a dinosaur. Is that a dream or a goal?

  (*Allow for responses.*)

- Right! That is a dream because it is not possible!
- OK, how about this one? I want to learn how to ride a unicycle. Is that a dream or a goal?

  (*Allow for responses.*)

- Right! That is a goal because it is possible, and I can learn to get good or better at it.
- How about this one: I want to learn how to hold my breath for three whole months! Is that a dream or a goal?

  (*Allow for responses.*)

- Right! That is a dream because it is not possible.
- Now that we understand what a goal is, it is important to know that since goals are about things that are possible and they are about things that you can get good or better at, the best goals always have plans and those are the kinds of goals we will be talking about today.

  (*Begin the session by starting a discussion about things that you as the counselor feel that you do well. You can say "I think I'm really good at drawing." Or you can say something like, "I think I'm really good at being kind." Try to make your examples relevant to the goals you wish the children to think of. At this time, draw three columns on the board, whiteboard or chart paper. Label the first one "I'm good at..." Label the second one "My goal for this year..." and label the third one "My plan..." Alternately, for nonreaders, draw a smiley face in column one, an archery target in column two and a smiley face with a thought bubble in the third column. For ease of use, you can also use the Goal Chart for Classrooms provided at the end of this chapter.*)

- What do you do really well?

  (*Allow for responses, then write or draw responses in the first column on the board, whiteboard or chart paper.*)

- It is great to know the things we are good at. It makes us feel really good! But having and reaching goals makes us feel really good too!
- How do you feel about these things that you do really well?

  (*Allow for responses.*)

- How did you learn how to do these things?

  (*Allow for responses.*)

- How did you get better at them?

  (*Allow for responses.*)

- Were these things hard to learn?

  (*Allow for responses.*)

- Did it take time or energy to learn how to do these things?

  (*Allow for responses.*)

- It is wonderful to know how to do things and feel proud about them. I am so happy that there are so many things you are all so good at! But what about things you are not good at yet? Are there any things you would like to get good at this year?

  (*Allow for responses.*)

- There are so many things that you want to become better at doing! If the things that you chose are possible and you can get better at doing them then they can be called goals. Let's write some of those goals on the board.

  (*Choose the responses that are viable goals. Try also to get the students to understand that the things that they choose should be realistic, attainable and just slightly difficult. If what they choose is too difficult, they may give up. If what they choose is too easy, it is not an appropriate goal to work toward. The goals could be life skills such as learning to tie their shoes or learning to swim, or they can be school goals such as learning to read better or to count by twos. Write or draw responses in the second column on the board, whiteboard or chart paper.*)

- These are all great ideas! But how do we get better at doing things? Do you remember when I said that I wanted to learn how to ride a unicycle? What are some things I can do so that I can learn how to ride it?

  (*Allow for responses. Choose responses that align with learning how to ride a unicycle. Choose responses such as "watch videos," "ask a friend to help" or "practice." Write or draw responses in the third column.*)

- The answers you gave are all part of a great way to learn how to ride a unicycle. Together, they make up my plan. If I ask people to help teach me and then I practice a little every day, do you think that this might be a good plan for me to learn how to ride a unicycle?

  (*Allow for responses.*)

- What might happen if I only had a goal, but I didn't have a plan?

  (*Allow for responses. Look for responses that lead the students toward understanding that in order to achieve goals, there must be steps, or a plan, in place to get there.*)

- Right! Sometimes if you have goals but no plan you might not be able to achieve that goal. Without a plan, that goal might be more a dream than a goal. Plans help us make our goals into things that can actually happen!

- What about you? Let's talk about your goals. Who can tell me a goal that they have for this year?

  (*Allow for responses. Lead students back to the responses in column two.*)

- Let's talk about your plans now. How are you going to achieve that goal?

  (*Allow for responses. Make sure that the students you call on restate their goal first and then tell their plan. Have several students give examples until it is clear that the students understand the concept.*)

- Those are all great ideas! I think we understand goals and plans a little better now. Now we will all get to figure out and work on our own personal plans.

  (*Hand out the worksheet 1.1. Make sure that students have pencils and/or crayons.*)

- Under the first question (My goal – What I want to get better at doing) write or draw a picture of one thing that you would like to get better at doing. Remember, we call this your "goal."

  (*Give students time to think about and then write or draw their responses.*)

- For the second question, we are going to write or draw our plan for getting better at our goal. What steps do we have to take to make sure that we can get better at our goal? Think about this question as you answer to the second question on the sheet.

  (*Allow students time to finish the worksheet.*)

- Now that we have finished our plans, I am going to place you into small groups so that we can share our goals and our plans. Remember that everyone should get a chance to share their goal and plan, and remember that while another person is talking, we stay respectful and quiet so that we can listen.

  (*When students have finished, place them into groups of two or three. Once the students are placed in groups, remind them that they are sharing their goals and plans. Make sure to walk around the room and give feedback as you hear their goals and the ideas for their plans. When the students have all finished sharing, bring them back to their regular seats.*)

- Does anyone want to share their goal or plan with the class?

  (*Allow for responses.*)

- Everyone did a great job today! We learned about goals and plans, and everyone came up with some wonderful ones. Remember that without a plan for reaching our goal, your goal becomes much harder to reach. Let's finish up with a few questions to make sure everyone understands. What is the difference between a goal and a dream?

  (*Allow for responses Make certain that the students understand that a goal is attainable and realistic and has a plan attached to it.*)

- What can happen if you don't have a plan for reaching your goal?

  (*Allow for responses. Make certain that the students understand that if the goal does not have a plan, then it might not be reached.*)

- What will you remember about today's lesson?

  (*Allow for responses.*)

If needed, enlarge the goal chart and use as the board example for nonreaders.

Student name:_____

Today's date:_____

Go for the Goal!

1.My goal - What I want to get better at doing.

_____

2.My plan - Ideas for getting better at doing it.

_____

_____

Handout 1.1

Things I Am Good At	Things I Want to Get Good At (My Goals)	My Plan

Worksheet 1.2 Goal Chart for Classroom

GOAL SETTING LESSON PLAN

Fourth to Fifth Grade

Materials:

> Whiteboard, chart paper or board
> Marker or chalk
> Handout 1.3 – Here I Goal!

Say the following:

- Today we will be discussing goal setting. Who can tell me the difference between a goal and a dream?

  (*Allow for responses.*)

- The difference between goals and dreams is that dreams can be about anything. You can dream that you want to be a basketball player, or you can dream that you want to discover the lost city of Atlantis. Goals, however, have to be possible and have to contain a plan to achieve them. So, for example, if I want a dinosaur as a pet, would that be a goal or a dream?

  (*Allow for responses, anticipating that students might say that it is a dream.*)

- Those of you who think it is a dream, tell me why you think it is a dream and not a goal.

  (*Allow for responses. Lead students to the idea that dinosaurs are extinct, so it is not possible to have a dinosaur as a pet.*)

- Right, so my desire to have a dinosaur as a pet is a dream because it is not possible. What if I wanted to be a pilot, would that be a goal or a dream?

  (*Allow for responses, anticipating that students might say that it is a goal.*)

- OK, but what if I had no plans or even an interest in taking flying lessons? Is my desire to become a pilot still a goal or is it something else then?

  (*Allow for responses. Guide students to the fact that without a viable plan, becoming a pilot without ever taking flying lessons is most likely a dream more than a goal.*)

- My desire to become a pilot is only realistic when I have a plan. Without any plans to actually learn how to fly a plane, this wish to become a pilot is more of a dream than a goal.
- The best goals always have plans and today we will be talking about those kinds of goals.

  (*Draw three columns on the whiteboard, chart paper or board. Label the first column "Things that I am already good at." Label the second column "My goal – Something that I would like to get better at doing." Label the third column "My plan – Ideas for getting better at doing it."*)

- Let's start with things we are already good at. Who wants to share something that they do well?

  (*Allow for responses and write these ideas on the chart or whiteboard under the first column, "Things that I am already good at." Make sure to focus on the ideas that require practice to perfect such as learning how to play a sport, learning to ride a bicycle or learning how to swim.*)

- How do you know you do these things well?

  (*Allow for responses.*)

- How did you learn how to do these things?

  (*Allow for responses.*)

- How did you get better at them?

  (*Allow for responses.*)

- Were these things hard to learn?

  (*Allow for responses.*)

- Did it take time or energy to learn how to do these things?

  (*Allow for responses.*)

- All of these things that you are already good at took work. You had to learn how to ride a bike or swim or read, and then you had to practice. Maybe you had to practice a little bit every night. Or maybe you set aside time every weekend. But all of the things you talked about are things that took work to improve or perfect. So now, let's look at things we are not good at yet. What are some things you might you like to work on or improve?

  (*Allow for responses. Try to get the children to choose things that interest them or to choose skills that they can improve. Try also to get them to understand that the things that they choose should be realistic, attainable and just slightly difficult. If what they choose is too difficult, they may give up. If what they choose is too easy, it is not an appropriate goal to work toward. Give examples such as getting better at math, getting better at reading or learning how to play soccer. Write the students' responses on the board under the second column "My goals – Something that I would like to get better at doing."*)

- These things that you want to get better at are called goals. Goals are things that are possible, realistic and take work to reach. Raise your hand if you think that you can learn to ride a bike by just closing your eyes and hoping that it happens.

  (*Allow for responses.*)

- Right! You can't just wish that things happen. You have to have a plan that you follow for making these things happen. So what is the plan for learning how to ride a bike?

  (*Allow for responses and make certain that the plan includes watching other people doing it, getting help from someone who knows how and practicing. Write the responses in the third column "My plan – Ideas for getting better at doing it."*)

- Concrete ideas to help reach your goals is the only way to reach goals. Just wanting to do something without taking any of the steps you need to get there is an example of a dream, not a goal. So someone who says that they want to become a professional football player but never practices is someone who just has a dream but not a goal. On the other hand, someone who wants to be a professional football player and they practice every day and find out how to get onto a professional team is someone who has a goal. What about someone who wants to do better in school? Is that a dream or is that a goal?

(*Allow for responses. Make sure that the students know that it could be either a dream or a goal dependent on the behavior of the student. If the student wants to do better in school but never hands in their homework, then their desire to be a better student is a dream. If, on the other hand, the student makes sure to study before every test, get help from their teachers and hands in every assignment, then this student's desire to become a better student is more of a goal than a dream.*)

• Now you will all create your own personal plans.

(*Give the students Handout 1.3 – Here I Goal! Have the students work individually to choose one thing they would like to get better at doing. Remind them that this is their "goal." Tell them that they will be writing this goal on the worksheet next to question number one "My goal – What I want to get better at doing." Tell the students that in the next column, "My plan – Ideas for getting better at doing it," they will be writing a few ideas of how to achieve their goal. Give the students time to fill in the worksheet. Make sure to walk around and see responses to give appropriate input.*)

• Now that you have filled in your worksheets, we are going to work with partners and share ideas. Make sure that each person in the group gets an opportunity to speak and make sure that every person listening is doing go respectfully and quietly.

(*Place the children into groups of two or three, and remind them that they are sharing their goals and the ideas for their plan with each other. Make sure each student gets a turn to share. Also make sure to walk around the room and give feedback as you hear their goals and the ideas for their plan.*)

• Let's pick someone from each group to share some of our goals and plans.

(*Have students choose a representative from each group to share their goals and plans.*)

• Everyone did such a good job understanding the difference between dreams and goals! Let's finish up with a few questions to make sure everyone understands. What can happen if you don't have a plan for reaching your goal?

(*Allow for responses and make sure that responses center on the idea that without a plan, you only have a dream, not a goal.*)

• What is the difference between a goal and a dream?

(*Allow for responses. Make certain that students understand that goals are concrete, attainable and realistic, while dreams can be about anything.*)

• What will you remember about today's lesson?

(*Allow for responses.*)

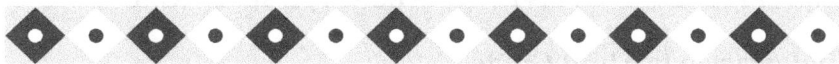

Student name:_____

Today's date:_____

Here I Goal!

1.My goal - What I want to get better at doing. (Write down one thing you would like to learn how to do better.)

_____

2.My plan - Ideas for getting better at doing it. What are some things you can do to help you reach your goal. Write down everything you can think of (even if you think it is silly!). Write on the back of this sheet if you need more room.

1._____   10._____

2._____   11._____

3._____   13._____

4._____   14._____

5._____   15._____

6._____   16._____

7._____   17._____

8._____   18._____

9._____   19._____

Handout 1.3

SELF-EFFICACY: POSITIVE AND NEGATIVE SELF-TALK

Kindergarten to Third Grade

Materials:

> Whiteboard, chart paper or board
> Marker or chalk
> Handout 2.1 – Mission to Planet Positive! Positive and Negative
>   Self-Talk
> Scissors
> Bag for garbage
> Pens or pencils for students

Say the following:

*   Last time we met we talked about goal setting. We talked about what goals were and how to achieve them, but having goals doesn't mean anything if you don't think that you can achieve them. Today, we will be talking about believing in ourselves. Raise your hand if you have ever had a hard time learning something new.

    (*Allow for responses.*)

*   That has happened to me too!

    (*Relate an experience of having a difficult time learning something new.*)

*   Raise your hand if while you were having a hard time learning something new, you started to feel bad about it.

    (*Allow for responses.*)

*   Me too!

    (*Relate how you felt about the thing you had a hard time learning how to do as well as the self-talk that kept you from reaching it. An example of this would be, "Once I wanted to learn how to speak Spanish. I tried really hard, but I just kept thinking that it was too hard so I gave up and felt really sad and disappointed in myself."*)

*   Has anyone here ever experienced something like that?

    (*Allow for responses and use questions to lead the students to discuss the incident itself as well as the feelings they experienced. Questions could be, What did you try to learn that was hard? How did you feel while you were trying to learn it?*)

*   One of the things I kept doing was telling myself that it was too hard. These things I was telling myself got in my way all the time! I kept telling myself that this was just too hard for me. When I started to

believe myself, that's when I gave up! Has anyone here ever had the experience of telling yourself that something is too hard and then you wanted to give up?

(*Allow for responses.*)

• This kind of talking to ourselves is called negative self-talk. Negative self-talk is when we tell ourselves bad things about ourselves. We might tell ourselves that we are not so smart or so capable or successful. Or we might tell ourselves that we are not tall enough or big enough or small enough. Whatever it is we tell ourselves with our negative self-talk, it makes us feel bad and it can change how successful we can be at things. We talk ourselves out of being successful! Has that experience ever happened it anyone in school with academic subjects?

(*Allow for responses.*)

• How did you feel about yourselves when that happened?

(*Allow for responses.*)

• Was there anything that you ever stopped doing or stopped trying as hard to do after you engaged in that negative self-talk?

(*Allow for responses.*)

• Who can give us some examples of the negative self-talk that you might have said to yourself?

(*Allow for responses. Use this question to make certain that the students understand what is meant by "negative self-talk" and gently correct as needed.*)

• So you see how destructive negative self-talk can be. It makes our ability to reach our goals so much harder to find. It may even keep us from achieving our goal completely! Today, our mission is to get rid of that negative self-talk. I am going to hand out a worksheet to each of you. Make sure that you have a pen or pencil and scissors because we are going to need them to work on the worksheet.

(*Distribute Handout 2.1 – Mission to Planet Positive! Hand out pens, pencils or scissors if needed. Pick up the worksheet and point to the column that is headed by the words "Negative Self-Talk."*)

• On this side of the worksheet, write down or draw any negative self-talk that has kept you or is keeping you from being successful in something. For example, you might have told yourself something like, "I'm just not good at math," or your negative self-talk might be, "Reading is so hard and I'm not good at it!" Whatever mean thing you tell yourself about you should go in this column. If you need more paper, raise your hand and I will bring you an extra worksheet. Please know that no one will be seeing these, not even me, so please let your statements be as honest as you can make them.

(Make sure that students are writing in the correct column. Allow students time to write down or draw their negative self-thoughts. Make certain everyone is done before proceeding. Also, make sure that you yourself have written some out as well.)

- Now, we are going to get rid of all of these mean thoughts about ourselves, but first we have to cut this part of the worksheet out. Let's take our scissors and cut out this whole column.

(Help students with cutting out the column if necessary.)

- Now, take the piece you have just cut out that is filled with all of those mean thoughts about yourself and we are going to crumble them into a ball! Imagine that you are crumbling your actual negative self-talk into that ball as well.

(Crumble your own column into a ball. Do it deliberately and decisively as a model for the students.)

- Now I am going to come around with a garbage bag and I want you to toss those thoughts away. I will do it as well!

(Toss your own negative thoughts column into the trash bag and walk around the room allowing each student to have a turn to toss their negative self-thoughts into the trash bag.)

- How does everyone feel?

(Allow for responses.)

- Great! But we are not done yet. Now we are going to replace those negative thoughts with positive ones. On the worksheet that should still be on your desk, there is one more column left. That column is titled "Positive Self-Talk." Just as negative self-talk can hurt us and keep us from being successful, positive self-talk can help us and lead us toward success. Positive self-talk is the nice things we say to ourselves in our heads. If I am doing positive self-talk, I will tell myself nice things. So, for example, if I am having trouble learning how to read, instead of telling myself that reading is too hard for me or that I am dumb and will never learn to read, I can tell myself that even if reading is hard, I am smart and I will learn to read eventually. Or maybe, instead of telling myself that I am bad at math, I can tell myself that even if math is hard and I am having a hard time right now, I will get it eventually. Can anyone give the class some examples of positive self-talk?

(Allow for responses. Make sure that students are including things such as, "I am smart enough to learn math" or "I am wonderful just as I am" or "I can learn to read better.")

- Yes, that is exactly what I mean by positive self-talk. We are going to use that column on the worksheet to write out or draw our own positive statements. If you have having trouble thinking of something, think of the things you wrote or drew as negative self-talk then write or draw the opposite. So, for example, if you wrote or drew that your negative self-talk was, "I am bad at math," then your positive self-talk can be, "I can be good at math." Write or draw your positive self-talk statements on your worksheet now.

  (*Allow time for the students to write or draw their positive self-talk statements on the worksheet. Make certain everyone has had a chance to finish before you move on.*)

- Does anyone want to share their positive self-talk statements with the group?

  (*Allow for responses and for sharing if necessary.*)

- You all did a great job. I want everyone to take these positive statements and place them somewhere they can stay with you for the whole year. Maybe you can place them in your pencil case or a folder. Wherever you choose to place them, make sure that you remove them from time to time and look at them to remind yourselves that you *can* achieve things and succeed.

  (*Allow time for students to store their worksheets.*)

- You all did such a good job throwing out your negative self-talk and replacing it with positive self-talk. Let's make sure that we keep all that negative self-talk away from us.
- Now, let's review everything we have learned. Who can tell the class what negative self-talk is?

  (*Allow for responses.*)

- Who can tell the class how negative self-talk can hurt us?

  (*Allow for responses.*)

- Who can tell the class what positive self-talk is?

  (*Allow for responses.*)

- Who can tell the class how positive self-talk can help us?

  (*Allow for responses.*)

- What is one thing you will remember from this class today?

  (*Allow for responses.*)

Name_____   Date_____

Mission to Planet Positive!

Positive and Negative Self-Talk

Negative Self-Talk	Positive Self-Talk
Mean things I tell myself about me	Nice things I tell myself about me

Handout 2.1

SELF-EFFICACY: POSITIVE AND NEGATIVE SELF-TALK

Fourth to Fifth Grade

Materials:

> Whiteboard, chart paper or board
> Marker or chalk
> Handout 2.2 – Positive and Negative Self-Talk: Talking to Ourselves
> Handout 2.3 – Tips for Keeping the Negative Thoughts Away
> Scissors
> Bag for garbage
> Pens or pencils for students

Say the following:

- Last time we met we talked about goal setting. We talked about what goals were and how to achieve them, but having goals doesn't mean anything if you don't believe that you can achieve them. In order to achieve your goals you have to believe that you can achieve them, so today we will be discussing how we can keep believing in our ability to achieve our goals. This belief is called self-efficacy, but just because we should believe in our ability to achieve our goals does not mean that we always do. Sometimes we have doubts that we can achieve them. Has anyone here ever had doubts about being able to achieve a goal?

  (*Allow for responses.*)

- That has happened to me too!

  (*Relate an experience of not having believed that you, the counselor, could reach a particular goal. Make certain that you relate the goal you were trying to reach, as well as the self-talk that kept you from reaching it. An example of this would be, "Once I wanted to learn how to speak Spanish. I tried really hard but I just kept thinking that it was too hard so I gave up."*)

- Has anyone here ever experienced something like that?

  (*Allow for responses.*)

- One of the things I kept doing was telling myself that it was too hard to do and that was what got in my way. There was this voice in my head – my voice – that kept telling me that it was just too hard for me. When I started to believe that voice, that's when I gave up! Has anyone here ever had the experience of telling yourself that something is too hard and then you gave up?

  (*Allow for responses.*)

- This kind of talking to ourselves is called negative self-talk. We tell ourselves that we can't do something and then we start to believe it. It can change how successful we can be at things. We talk ourselves out of being successful! Has that experience ever happened to anyone in school with academic subjects?

   (*Allow for responses.*)

- How did you feel about yourselves when that happened?

   (*Allow for responses.*)

- Was there anything that you ever stopped doing or stopped trying as hard to do after you engaged in that negative self-talk?

   (*Allow for responses.*)

- So you see how destructive negative self-talk can be. It makes our self-efficacy, or our belief in our ability to reach our goals, harder to find. It may even make it disappear completely. But today we are going to get rid of that negative self-talk. I am going to hand out a worksheet to each of you. Make sure that you have a pen or pencil and scissors because we are going to need them.

   (*Distribute the worksheet. Hand out pens, pencils or scissors if needed. Pick up the worksheet and point to the column that is headed by the words "Negative Self-Talk."*)

- On this side of the worksheet, write down or draw any negative self-talk that has kept you or is keeping you from being successful in something. For example, you might have told yourself something like, "I'm just not good at math," or your negative self-talk might be, "Reading is so hard! I'm not doing this reading right now. I'll get to it eventually." But then you never get back to it! If you need more paper, raise your hand and I will bring you an extra worksheet. Please know that no one will be seeing these, not even me, so please let your statements be as honest as you can make them. If you would like, your worksheet can have any other negative thoughts about yourself that you have had. Some examples of this might be that sometimes we think we are not enough of something to be worthwhile – not tall enough, not thin enough, not smart enough. Whatever your negative self-talk is, write down or draw each one in the box underneath the heading "Negative Self-Talk."

   (*Make sure that students are writing in the correct column. Allow students time to write down or draw their negative self-thoughts. Make certain everyone is done before proceeding. Also, make sure that you yourself have written some out as well.*)

- Now, we are going to take the scissors and cut out this whole column.

  (*Help students with cutting out the column if necessary.*)

- Now, take your column filled with all of those negative thoughts and crumble them into a ball! Imagine that you are crumbling your actual negative self-talk into that ball as well.

  (*Crumble your own column into a ball. Do it deliberately and decisively as a model for the students.*)

- Now I am going to come around with a garbage bag and I want you to toss those thoughts away. I will do it as well!

  (*Toss your own negative thoughts column into the trash bag and walk around the room allowing each student to have a turn to toss their negative self-thoughts into the trash bag.*)

- How does everyone feel?

  (*Allow for responses.*)

- Great! But we are not done yet. Now we are going to replace those negative thoughts with positive ones. On the worksheet that should still be on your desk, there is one more column left. That column is titled "Positive Self-Talk." Just as negative self-talk can hurt us and keep us from being successful, positive self-talk can help us and lead us toward success. Can anyone tell the class what I might mean by positive self-talk?

  (*Allow for responses. Make sure that students are including things such as, "I am smart enough to learn math" or "I am wonderful just as I am" or "I can learn to read better."*)

- Yes, that is exactly what I mean by positive self-talk. We are going to use that column on the worksheet to write out or draw our own positive statements. If you are having trouble thinking of something, think of the things you wrote or drew as negative self-talk then write or draw the opposite. So, for example, if you wrote or drew that your negative self-talk was "I am bad at math," then your positive self-talk can be "I can be good at math." Write or draw your positive self-talk statements on your worksheet now.

  (*Allow time for the students to write or draw their positive self-talk statements on the worksheet. Make certain everyone has had a chance to finish before you move on.*)

- Does anyone want to share their positive self-talk statements with the group?

  (*Allow for responses and for sharing if necessary.*)

- You all did a great job. I want everyone to take these positive statements and place them somewhere they can stay with you for the whole year. Maybe you can place them in your pencil case or a folder. Wherever you choose to place them, make sure that you remove them from time to time and reread them to remind yourselves that you *can* achieve things and succeed.

  (*Allow time for students to store their worksheets.*)

- You all did such a good job throwing out your negative self-talk and replacing it with positive self-talk. Let's make sure that we keep all that negative self-talk away from us.

  (*Hand out Handout 2.3 – Tips for Keeping the Negative Thoughts Away. Review the handout with the class and answer any questions as needed.*)

- Great! I want you to keep this handout someplace safe as well and refer back to as often as you need to. Now, let's review everything we have learned. Who can tell the class what negative self-talk is?

  (*Allow for responses.*)

- Who can tell the class how negative self-talk can hurt us?

  (*Allow for responses.*)

- Who can tell the class one way to keep negative thoughts away?

  (*Allow for responses.*)

- Who can tell the class what positive self-talk is?

  (*Allow for responses.*)

- Who can tell the class how positive self-talk can help us?

  (*Allow for responses.*)

- What is one thing you will remember from this class today?

  (*Allow for responses.*)

Name_____   Date_____

Positive and Negative Self-Talk
Talking to Ourselves!

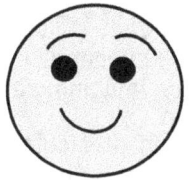

Negative Self-Talk	Positive Self-Talk
What negative things do I tell myself that keep me from being my best?	What positive things do I tell myself that help me be my best?

Handout 2.2

Name_____ Date_____

Tips for Keeping the Negative Thoughts Away

1. Think about a time you DID succeed!
    Remembering or even imagining a success helps to make it happen again!
2. Ask for help when things get difficult.
    No one likes to admit that things are difficult for them but if you don't ask for help, you will still need help anyway, you just won't get it!
3. Stay positive.
    Keep things upbeat and don't fall into negative thinking.
4. Surround yourself with good friends.
    Make sure you have friends who make you feel good about what you can do.
5. Don't allow setbacks to make you quit.
    Admit the setback and find a way around it - "I couldn't remember what came after the letter N! I bet if I start over, I might remember." And if you still can't, ask for help.
6. Copy what successful students do.
    If your friend is always getting good grades, ask them what they do to make that happen and follow their example.
7. Change your behavior.
    If you studied for a test and did not do well, don't give up. Just try a different way of studying next time.

Handout 2.3

SELF-REGULATION: ANGER

Kindergarten to Third Grade

Materials:

> Handout 3.1 – These Things Bug Me!
> Handout 3.2 – Bugs, Bugs Go Away! Positive Ways to Handle My Anger
> Pencils
> Crayons
> Plastic bugs – enough to hand out three or four to each student
> Whiteboard, chart paper or board
> Marker or chalk

Say the following:

- Today we are going to talk about being angry and what we can do about it. Raise your hand if you have ever been angry.

  (*Allow for responses.*)

- What kinds of things get you angry?

  (*Allow for responses.*)

- Everyone has things that bother them. Some things bug us so much that we don't know what to do with them. It is OK to be angry, but sometimes being angry gets in our way and keeps us from doing the things we need to do. One time, I got so angry at my friend that I did not talk to them for a long time and even missed their birthday party! Has anyone ever been angry and missed out on something because of it?

  (*Allow for responses.*)

- It sounds like we have all had that experience. Today we will be talking about things that bug us and what we can do about it. Something that bugs us is something that bothers us or makes us feel angry. I will be handing out a bunch of bugs to each one of you. Don't worry they're all plastic. Each one of the bugs will represent something that bothers you or makes you angry.

  (*Hand out several plastic bugs per student.*)

- Now look at the bugs in front of you and think of something that bugs you. Pick up one of the bugs and think about what bugs you. What bugs you?

  (*Ask each student and allow them to share one thing that makes them upset or angry. Go around the group members until everyone who wants to share has shared.*)

- We can get upset or bothered about lots of different things. I am bugged when I can't find my keys in the morning. I am also bugged when someone takes something of mine without asking. I want you to pick up a bug and bring it closer to you for each thing that bothers you and makes you angry. Don't worry if you have more things that bug you than you have bugs. We are only going to talk about a few of the things that bug you, not all of them. While you pick your bugs, I am going to hand out a handout.

   (*Hand out Handout 3.1 – These Things Bug Me!*)

- Once you have your bugs and your handout, I want you to think about those things that bug you. On the handout, write or draw a picture of each of those things that bug you, that means that you should write down each thing that makes you angry or upset.

   (*Give students enough time to write or draw the things that make them angry or upset.*)

- Let's share what we have come up with. Who wants to go first?

   (*Give time for students to volunteer their answers.*)

- Now that we know what bugs us, what are we going to do about it? How do we handle it when we get upset or angry? Some things that help me when I am angry are going on a walk, taking a warm bath or talking to a good friend. What about you? What helps you when you are angry or upset?

   (*Have students volunteer things to do to deal with anger. Lead students toward productive and positive ideas and write these on the board.*)

- Excellent! You have all come up with some great ways to handle your anger! I'm going to hand out another handout and we will use that handout to write or draw the positive ways we can deal with our anger.

   (*Hand out Handout 3.2 – Bugs, Bugs Go Away! Positive Ways to Handle My Anger. Give students enough time to complete the handout.*)

- Who wants to share some of the positive things that they can do to handle their anger?

   (*Allow students to share their positive ways of handling their anger.*)

- Is it OK to be angry?

   (*Allow for responses.*)

- Is it OK to be angry if it causes you to miss things or do things that you might regret later?

   (*Allow for responses.*)

- What are some positive things you can do when you are angry in order to help you feel better?

  (*Allow for responses.*)

- You all did a wonderful job learning about being angry and managing your anger. What is one thing you will remember from today's lesson?

  (*Allow for responses.*)

Name_____   Date_____

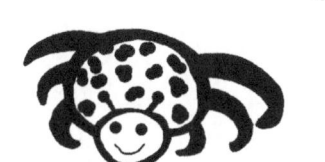

1.

2.

3.

4.

Handout 3.1

Name_____   Date_____

Bugs, Bugs Go Away!
Positive Ways to Handle My Anger

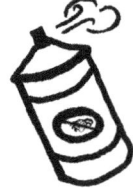

1.

2.

3.

4.

Handout 3.2

SELF-REGULATION: ANGER

Fourth to Fifth Grade

Materials:

> Handout 3.3 – My Best Choices
> Pens, pencils
> Handout 3.4 – Scenarios (each scenario should be cut out)

Say the following:

- Raise your hand if you have ever felt like anger sometimes takes over and makes you lose control. Put your hands down.
- Raise your hand if you have ever acted impulsively based on anger. Put your hands down.
- Raise your hand if you have ever felt better or less stressed out after you have taken your anger out on another person or thing. Put your hands down.
- Raise your hand if you have ever acted on your anger without thinking. Put your hands down.
- Raise your hand if you have ever regretted some of the choices or decisions you have made based on anger. Put your hands down.
- There are times when everyone lets their anger get the best of them and it affects their ability to make good judgments. Sometimes it is hard to think before we react, and this might lead us to say or do things that we regret. This can happen to anyone. I have had times when it has happened to me as well.

(Share a time that it has happened to you, the counselor.)

- Sometimes, when we lose control to anger, it has some negative consequences. For example, if I get really angry and throw something, it can break and then I might feel upset that I broke it. Or maybe, if I get really angry and I yell at someone, even if I don't mean it or I'm sorry immediately, they might be really mad at me and might not want to be friends with me anymore. What are some other negative things that can happen when you lose control of your anger?

(Allow for responses.)

- Has anyone experienced anything negative that was a result of you losing control of your anger?

(Allow for responses.)

- Who can share an instance when this has happened?

(Allow for responses.)

- So we see how important it is to keep our anger in check. Lots of bad things can happen when we don't. Today we are going to work on how to manage our anger in positive ways. We are going to start by looking at some smart choices and good alternatives to letting anger get the best of us.

(*Hand out Handout 3.3 – My Best Choices.*)

- This handout has some really good alternatives to letting anger take over. Let's look at some of these smart choices for dealing with our anger.

  (*Review the alternatives to acting on anger on Handout 3.3.*)

- Why do you think it is important to have alternatives to letting our anger take control of us?

  (*Allow for responses.*)

- Let's take a minute while you all choose which of these things might be helpful for you. Circle the ones you think will help you. How do you think this might help?

  (*Allow for responses.*)

- When do you think that you might use this?

  (*Allow for responses.*)

- Can you think of some other ideas that might help you keep your anger at bay?

  (*Allow for responses.*)

- Let's take a minute and write or draw those ideas on the bottom of your sheet.

  (*Allow time for students to write or draw other ideas for alternatives to acting out on anger.*)

- Now we are going to get to practice these great alternatives to letting anger get the best of us. I am going to hand each group a different sheet of paper with a scenario that might cause someone to be angry. I will help you read it if you need me to, but first, I am going to separate you into small groups.

  (*Separate the students into small groups. Make sure that all of the scenarios from Handout 3.4 have been cut individually and hand out one scenario to each group.*)

- You have two jobs that need to be done. Your first job is to decide what the person in the scenario is feeling. Your second job is to use your smart choices list and come up with a way for your character to deal with this situation without resorting to anger.

  (*Give the students a few minutes to review the scenario and come up with appropriate and positive responses.*)

- You all did a wonderful job. I am going to let you pick one member of your group to present to the class. Remember that we are first identifying the feeling the character is feeling and then tell the best strategy for that situation.

  (Allow each group to present. Make sure to lead them to identifying the feeling, telling the best strategy and then ask the group why this strategy was chosen.)

- You guys did a great job! It is important to know that we have choices about how we handle our feelings. So let's take some time to review.
- What are some negative things that can happen when we give into our anger?

  (Allow for responses.)

- What are some good alternatives to giving in to our anger?

  (Allow for responses.)

- How can these alternatives help you?

  (Allow for responses.)

- What is one thing you will remember about today's lesson?

  (Allow for responses.)

Name_____   Date_____

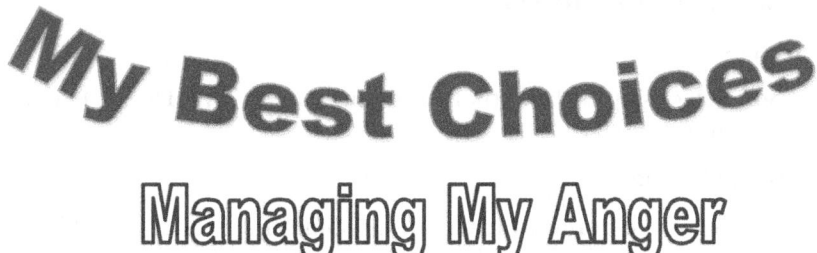

My Best Choices
Managing My Anger

1. Journal it ✏
2. Talk to someone 👥
3. Move around
4. Listen to music ♪

My own choices...

Handout 3.3

Handout 3.4 – Scenarios

1. During recess, your best friend tells you that they don't want to play with you because you were mean to them earlier. You don't have any idea what they are talking about and don't remember being mean, but when you try to explain, they tell you that they don't care and then walk away.
2. You are the only one out of your group of friends who was not invited to go with them to the mall. Each time you try to find out when they are going, they all ignore you.
3. You find out that your sister has been reading your diary and telling her friends about what you have written.
4. The student behind you stole your pen. You try to tell the teacher, but he only says that you need to be doing your work right now and not worrying about other people.
5. You think that your friend has been spreading rumors about you. One day, you see a group of students sitting with your friend and they all seem to be looking in your direction and laughing.
6. You studied for a test for a long time but failed it anyway.
7. Your teacher tells you that she is surprised that you did all of your homework for a change.

ATTENDING

Kindergarten to Third Grade

Materials:

> Soft bell or singing bowl (bell must maintain its sound for an extended time)

Say the following:

*   Today we are going to learn about something called mindfulness. Does anyone know what the word "mindfulness" means?

    (*Allow for responses.*)

*   Mindfulness is the act of making your mind focus on what is happening right now. Can anyone tell me something that is happening right now?

    (*Allow for responses and lead as necessary.*)

*   Those are all things that are happening right now. You were being mindful when you were listening for them. Being mindful means that we are paying close attention to the things that are happening right now instead of thinking about the things that might happen. Using

mindfulness can help us learn to focus, or pay attention, better, to find our calmness if we are angry, to deal with things in a calm way if we are nervous, and to find our way to peaceful thoughts when we are sad or frustrated. Why might it be important to learn to focus, or pay attention better?

(Allow for responses, but lead the students toward the idea that learning is more effective when students can pay attention and focus.)

- Right! Why might it be important to stay calm if we are angry?

  (Allow for responses, but lead the students toward the idea that people who are angry might make poor decisions.)

- Great answers! Why might it be important to find peaceful thoughts is we are sad or frustrated?

  (Allow for responses, but lead the students toward the idea that feeling too sad or frustrated could get in the way of learning or enjoying themselves.)

- That's right! All of your answers are so great! I think it might be time to practice some mindfulness right now! Let's try it right now for a minute. I want everyone to pay attention to the things you are hearing. Try to focus on the sounds. For example, if I stay very quiet, I can hear the birds chirping outside or sounds of other children in other classrooms. We are going to sit mindfully in a short while, but first I have a question for you. Do you think that you can hear the sounds of the birds chirping outside if you are making noise?

  (Allow for responses.)

- Right. That means that in order to do this exercise in mindfulness, we are going to have to be very, very quiet. So for the next few minutes, you are going to sit very quietly and see if you can hear the sounds of the birds chirping outside or any other sound you might hear, but remember, if you are making noise, you might not hear it. So for the next few minutes, we are going to sit very quietly and just listen. We will stay quietly listening until I play this sound (play the soft bell or singing bowl). Ready? Let's start right now.

  (Allow one or two minutes of silence. If the group is young, or if they have trouble focusing, don't make the silence last too long.)

- What did you hear?

  (Allow for responses. Make sure that the responses are all focused on things that the students actually heard during the time they were quiet.)

- Those are all great sounds you heard! While you were so busy listening to what was going on right in those minutes, you might have been too focused on listening to have been thinking about anything else. You might have been too busy focusing on what was going on in those minutes to worry about homework or friends. You might have been too busy focusing on what was going on in those minutes to think about anything that might happen in the future or anything that has already happened in the past.

- You all did a great job! Was that hard or easy?

(Allow for responses.)

- OK, we are going to do this again, but this time we are going to do this a little bit differently. I am going to ring the bell again and I want you to listen to it until you can't hear it anymore. I am going to show you what I mean. I will ring it now and I want you to listen carefully and raise your hand when you don't hear the sound anymore.

(Ring bell and wait for the students to raise their hands at the end of the sound.)

- Good job! This time we are going to close our eyes and also try to keep very still, and then I will ring the bell. When I ring the bell a second time, that is when we will all open our eyes. Keeping still and keeping our eyes closed helps us concentrate on these mindful sounds we are trying to hear. Keep your eyes closed, keep as still as you can and here we go.

(Ring the bell, wait for the sound to end and ring the bell again.)

- Great job! How did that feel? How many of you were able to hear the bell all the way to the end?

(Allow for responses.)

- You are all getting very good at this! We are going to try this one more time and this time we are going to put it all together. This time, while we are all sitting very still and keeping our eyes closed, I will ring the bell and you will listen to the bell all the way to the end, and then also listen to whatever sounds you hear that are not the bell sound. Just like before, we will open our eyes once we hear the start of the second bell. Try to pay attention to loud sounds and soft sounds. Try to hear the softest sound you can hear and pay close attention to all of the sounds you hear. Let's close our eyes and make ourselves comfortable in our chairs.

(Give students a chance to get comfortable and then ring the bell and begin. Try to have the children stay mindful and quiet for longer than the time before – at least a full minute.)

- You all did great! Raise your hand to share some loud sounds you might have heard.

(Allow for responses.)

- Raise your hand to share some soft sounds you might have heard.

  (*Allow for responses.*)

- You all did such a great job hearing loud and soft sounds. Raise your hand if you think that you had to sit very quietly in order to hear some of those soft sounds.

  (*Allow for responses.*)

- It is true. You had to sit very quiet to hear some of those soft sounds. What was the softest sound you heard?

  (*Allow for responses.*)

- Those are some of the sounds I heard too! Letting ourselves sit quietly and listening is a way of learning how to pay attention. Sometimes it is hard to pay attention, but when you practice doing it, it becomes easier and easier. Try to listen to all of those soft sounds for the rest of the day and let me know what you hear.
- Let's finish this lesson by answering a few questions. What is one way of being mindful?

  (*Allow for responses, but lead students to the response of "sitting quietly and listening."*)

- Why do we need to sit quietly to listen mindfully?

  (*Allow for responses, but lead students to the idea that quiet listening lets you hear things you might not otherwise hear.*)

- What is one thing you will remember from today?

  (*Allow for responses.*)

ATTENDING

Fourth to Fifth Grade

Materials:

> A long string – About one and one half to two feet long, with a small weight (such as a washer) tied to the bottom of it. Enough for each student to have one.
> Handout 4.1 – Changing Our Self-Talk
> Pens or pencils for writing

Say the following:

- Even if we don't want to admit it, everyone talks to themselves every single day. We might not talk to ourselves out loud, but we are constantly telling ourselves things. For example, on my way in to work this morning, I realized that I forgot my lunch. I got really upset about it and told myself, "You are so dumb! How could you forget your lunch? It was right on the counter and now it is going to be garbage because it's been out all day." How do you think I made myself feel when I called myself "dumb"?

(*Allow for responses.*)

- Definitely. I made myself feel pretty bad. And even though I know that I am not dumb, I felt pretty dumb and that is not a good feeling at all! Has anyone ever talked to themselves like that?

(*Allow for responses.*)

- How did it make you feel?

(*Allow for responses.*)

- What about when you talk to yourself while you are doing something that is difficult? I recently have been trying to teach myself computer coding (or whatever you, the counselor, are comfortable saying). It is super hard, and it takes a lot of concentration and focus. Last week, when I just could not get it right, I said to myself, "This is too hard. I am never going to be able to learn this. Why am I doing this anyway? Maybe I am just not smart enough to be able to understand this stuff. I think I might just give up." Has anyone ever done any talking to themselves like this?

(*Allow for responses.*)

- How did this make you feel?

(*Allow for responses.*)

- Did anyone give up trying something because of those thoughts?

(*Allow for responses.*)

- We all talk to ourselves about lots of different things all the time. What are some other things that we might say to ourselves?

(*Allow for responses.*)

- How do those things make you feel? How is your behavior affected by those things?

(*Allow for responses.*)

- What we tell ourselves is incredibly powerful. It affects us in ways that we might not even know. In fact, I'm going to show you how talking to yourself might affect you.

(*Hand one string with small weight attached to it to each student.*)

- Everyone should have a string with a little weight attached to the end. I want everyone to stand up and hold the string up in front of them like this.

  (*Demonstrate holding the string while dangling the small weight at the end of it.*)

- Now tell yourself what direction you want the washer to move in, but don't actively try to make it move.

  (*Give time for students to engage in the activity.*)

- What happened?

  (*Allow for responses.*)

- Why do you think that happened?

  (*Allow for responses.*)

- The things we tell ourselves are incredibly powerful in ways we might not even be aware of. Many times, the things we tell ourselves are negative thoughts. Things like, "I hate writing" or "I hate math" or "I'm not good at reading." These negative thoughts have an impact on our behavior whether we know it or not. Just like the washer, telling ourselves these negative things might make negative behavior happen. What kinds of negative things do you tell yourself?

  (*Allow for responses.*)

- How do these thoughts translate into behavior?

  (*Allow for responses.*)

- Does anyone ever tell themselves anything positive like, "You are doing a great job learning how to write better" or "You are really starting to understand long division!"

  (*Allow for responses.*)

- For some reason it seems a lot easier to beat ourselves up and convince ourselves of the negative stuff than it is to tell ourselves anything positive. Since we know that what we tell ourselves has an impact on us, and we know that telling ourselves negative things can have a negative impact, what can telling ourselves positive things do for us?

  (*Allow for responses.*)

- Let's try this together. Who wants to share some difficult task that they have recently had to do? Perhaps it was a really hard homework assignment or maybe it was learning some brand-new concept in school. Who wants to share what that difficult thing was for them?

  (*Allow for responses.*)

- Think back to that moment. What kinds of things were you telling yourself while you were trying to accomplish that task?

  (*Allow for responses.*)

- What was the end result of that task?

  (*Allow for responses.*)

- What if instead of just letting that negative self-talk, we were able to take a minute, hear those thoughts but replace them with positive self-talk instead? For example, if I am having a hard time learning division maybe I will take a minute and ask myself what that script in my head sounds like. Maybe during that time, I realize that I have been telling myself that I am just not that smart and that math is too hard. Once I take that minute and hear the negative self-talk, I can easily replace it with something else. What can I tell myself instead?

  (*Allow for responses.*)

- Right. I can tell myself all of those things. I can even tell myself honestly that yes, I am having a hard time understanding this concept, but just because I don't get it today, doesn't mean that I still won't understand it at another point. Maybe I can change what I tell myself to something like, "I don't get this … yet." This way, I am being honest about how hard it is but also not letting myself think that I will never understand it. Let's try to change that negative self-talk to positive self-talk together.

  (*Hand out Handout 4.1 – Changing Our Self-Talk.*)

- Everyone read along while I read the directions out loud.

  (*Read the directions aloud.*)

- Let's take a few minutes and complete the handout. I will come around to each of you to help you.

  (*Give the students a few minutes to finish their handouts. Make sure to walk around the classroom checking work and helping as needed.*)

- Great! Who wants to share their answer to the first scenario?

  (*Allow for responses.*)

- How could the negative self-talk have hurt here?

  (*Allow for responses.*)

- How could the positive self-talk help?

  (*Allow for responses.*)

- Excellent work. You all did a great job changing negative self-talk into positive self-talk. Who wants to remind us of why it is important to take a minute and ask ourselves what we are telling ourselves while we are doing something difficult?

  (*Allow for responses.*)

- How can negative self-talk hurt us?

  (*Allow for responses.*)

- How can positive self-talk help us?

  (*Allow for responses.*)

- What is one thing you will remember about this lesson?

  (*Allow for responses.*)

Handout 4.1 – Changing Our Self-Talk

Read the following scenarios:

- Write or think about what might happen because of the negative self-talk.
- Change the negative self-talk into positive self-talk.
- Write or think about what might happen because of the positive self-talk.
  1. Your teacher returns a test that you studied very hard for. When you look at the grade, you see that you failed it.
     Negative self-talk: I am stupid, and this proves it. I will never be able to do well on this!
     What might happen now: _____
     _____
     Positive self-talk: _____
     _____
     What might happen now: _____
     _____

  2. You are given a reading assignment for homework and reading takes you a long time.
     Negative self-talk: I hate reading. I am so bad at it!
     What might happen now: _____
     _____
     Positive self-talk: _____
     _____
     What might happen now: _____
     _____

MEMORY

Kindergarten to Third Grade

Materials:

> Large and labeled map of classroom to place on floor
> Markers or chalk
> Printed pictures of the following (the size of the pictures should be
>   able to fit into spaces of the map):
> Carrots
> Horse
> Dog
> Cat
> Cow
> Pickle
> Pencil
> Phone
> Baby

Say the following:

- How many of you have ever had trouble remembering things?

  (*Allow for responses.*)

- What kinds of things do you have trouble remembering?

  (*Allow for responses.*)

- I have trouble remembering things sometimes too. I have trouble remembering appointments, what I need to buy at the grocery store, birthdays and lots of other things too, but I found a secret and I am going to share it with you. My secret is called mnemonics. Has anyone ever heard that word before?

  (*Allow for responses.*)

- Mnemonics is a big word that refers to a system you might use to help you remember things, but we are going to call these things "memory tricks." In fact, you might even use memory tricks right now and don't even know it. How many of you know the colors of the rainbow?

  (*Allow for responses.*)

- How do you remember them in order?

  (*Allow for responses and lead students to the mnemonic "ROY G BIV," which stands for red, orange, yellow, green, blue, indigo and violet. If students do not know it, write it out on the board with the words beneath and make sure to say each word aloud.*)

- ROY G BIV is a memory trick which allows us to remember colors of the rainbow, but there are lots of other ways to remember things too. Today we are going to learn a memory trick that uses something called visualization. Does anyone know what the word "visualization" means?

  (*Allow for responses.*)

- To visualize something means to see it in your head. Let's do a quick exercise to see what this looks like. Everybody close your eyes. I am going to say a word and I want you to try to see it in your head with your eyes closed. Ready? The word is tree. Remember, with your eyes closed I want you to see a tree.

  (*Give the students a few seconds to try to visualize a tree.*)

- Did everyone see it?

  (*Allow for responses.*)

- What did your tree look like?

  (*Allow for responses.*)

- Great. You guys did a wonderful job visualizing trees with your eyes closed. Today we are going to try to use memory tricks and visualization to remember a list of things in a way that may be new to many of you. We are going to start by hearing a list of things that I want you to remember. Here we go:
  Carrots
  Horse
  Dog
  Cat
  Cow
  Pickle
  Pencil
  Phone
  Baby
- Who can repeat the list back to me in the correct order?

  (*Allow for responses.*)

- Remembering things can be really hard but by using our memory tricks, we can make it a little easier.

  (*Repeat list, but this time show the students the pictures of the items as you say them.*)

- Now who can remember the list of items in the correct order?

  (*Allow for responses.*)

- Maybe seeing those pictures made it a little bit easier to remember the list but let's make it even easier.

  (*Clear an area on the floor for the large, labeled map of the classroom. Have the students sit around the map. Explain the map to the students and point out all of the areas of the classroom that you have labeled on the map. Make sure that there are at least nine separate areas that are clearly marked on the map. For example, there might be a reading corner, an art space, the door, the teachers desk, etc. Point things out in the order in which they appear on the map, starting at the door and going counterclockwise.*)

- We are going to take each one of these pictures and place each one in a different area of the classroom.

  (*Call a student to come up to the map and place the first picture from the list, the carrots, by the first area, which would be the door.*)

- We put the carrots in the area by the door. Can everyone see that?

  (*Repeat the procedure until all nine items have been placed in different areas of the map.*)

- Who can tell us where the carrots are?

  (*Allow students to look at the map to answer the question.*)

- That is right! The carrots are by the door! That is a silly place for carrots!

  (*Continue asking the students where each item is on the map until each item has been reviewed.*)

- Who can tell us what item is by the door?

  (*Allow for responses. The point of this is to solidify the images and their place in the map. Continue asking the students what item is in each area until all of the items have been reviewed*).

- Now we are going to make this a little bit more difficult. Everyone close your eyes.

  (*Remove one item from the map.*)

- Now open your eyes. Which item is missing?

  (*Allow for responses.*)

- Everyone close your eyes again. How about now? What two items are missing?

  (*Allow for responses. Repeat the procedure until all of the items have been removed.*)

• Now that all of the items have been removed, let's try to remember where everything went. I will start at the door and point to each area and you all tell me what item was there. Ready?

(*Point to the door on the map. The students should be able to tell you that the carrots were at the door. Continue pointing to each area until all of the items are mentioned.*)

• Wow! Look at that! You all used a memory trick to remember that long list of things that you might not have been able to remember otherwise. You all did such a great job remembering! Sometimes we can remember things just because we remember them, but other times it helps to use our memory tricks like we did today. Now we are going to finish our lesson with just one question. What do you think you are going to remember about today's lesson?

(*Allow for responses.*)

MEMORY

Fourth to Fifth Grade

Materials:

    Large and labeled map of classroom to place on floor
    Markers or chalk
    Printed pictures of the following (the size of the pictures should be able to fit into spaces of the map):
    Carrots
    Horse
    Dog
    Cat
    Cow
    Pickle
    Pencil
    Phone
    Baby

Say the following:

• How many of you have ever had trouble remembering things?

(*Allow for responses.*)

• What kinds of things do you have trouble remembering?

(*Allow for responses.*)

- I have trouble remembering things sometimes too. I have trouble remembering appointments, what I need to buy at the grocery store, birthdays and lots of other things too, but I found a secret and I am going to share it with you. My secret is called mnemonics. Has anyone ever heard that word before?

  (*Allow for responses.*)

- Mnemonics is a big word that refers to a system you might use to help you remember things, but we are going to call these things "memory tricks." In fact, you might even use memory tricks right now and don't even know it. How many of you know the colors of the rainbow?

  (*Allow for responses.*)

- How do you remember them in order?

  (*Allow for responses and lead students to the mnemonic "ROY G BIV," which stands for red, orange, yellow, green, blue, indigo and violet. If students do not know it, write it out on the board with the words beneath and make sure to say each word aloud.*)

- ROY G BIV is a memory trick that allows us to remember colors of the rainbow, but there are lots of other ways to remember things too. Today we are going to learn a memory trick that uses something called visualization. Does anyone know what the word visualization means?

  (*Allow for responses.*)

- To visualize something means to see it in your head. Let's do a quick exercise to see what this looks like. Everybody close your eyes. I am going to say a word and I want you to try to see it in your head with your eyes closed. Ready? The word is tree. Remember, with your eyes closed I want you to see a tree.

  (*Give the students a few seconds to try to visualize a tree.*)

- Did everyone see it?

  (*Allow for responses.*)

- What did your tree look like?

  (*Allow for responses.*)

- Great. You guys did a wonderful job visualizing trees with your eyes closed. Today we are going to try to use memory tricks and visualization to remember a list of things in a way that may be new to many of you. We are going to start by hearing a list of things that I want you to remember. Here we go:
  Carrots
  Horse
  Dog

Cat
Cow
Pickle
Pencil
Phone
Baby

- Who can repeat the list back to me in the correct order?

  (*Allow for responses.*)

- Remembering things can be really hard, but by using our memory tricks, we can make it a little easier. Remember a few minutes ago when I had you visualize a tree? I am going to repeat each item again, but I am going to repeat them slowly and give you some time to visualize the item in your mind before I move on to the next item. Are we ready?

  (*Repeat the list and give the students time to visualize each item before you move on. If needed, remind students that they are visualizing each item.*)

- Now who can remember the list of items in the correct order?

  (*Allow for responses.*)

- Maybe visualizing those images in our minds made it a little bit easier to remember the list, but let's make it even easier. We are going to do some more visualization. I am going to help you visualize a house. It could be your house or it could be someone's house that you know, but I want it to be something that you are familiar with and can see when you close your eyes. I want you to close your eyes and imagine walking into this place. You are opening the door and stepping inside. I want you to see the door as clearly as you can. Look at what the door is made of, look at the floor, the doorknob. I just want you to see it as well as you can. From here we are going to walk into the kitchen. We're going to stop in the doorway of the kitchen and look around. Look at the floor, look at the walls, look at all of the appliances. Now I want you to visualize walking toward the refrigerator. I want you to visualize standing in front of the refrigerator. I want you to look at the color of the refrigerator, I want you to look at the doors of the refrigerator, I want you to see everything that you possibly can about the refrigerator. Now let's walk toward the sink. Look at the sink carefully. Is it a deep sink? A shallow sink? What color is the sink? See as much of it as you can see. Now we will walk toward the cabinet to grab a glass. I want you to visualize opening that cabinet and grabbing a glass off the shelf. Look at the cabinet and see what it is made of or what kinds of knobs or pulls are on the outside of it. I want you to walk back to the sink and turn on the water to fill the cup. I want you to visualize the water coming out of the tap. I want you to look at it carefully and see what it looks like, what it sounds like. Could everyone see it?

(Allow for responses. If students have a difficult time visualizing, use the same lesson plan that was used for kindergarten to grade three.)

Now you walk toward your bedroom. Look at the room carefully. See the colors the walls are painted, look around at the stuff inside of it. You walk to your computer or TV and see it carefully. You can see the color of it, how big it is, you can even feel what it feels like. Finally, you are going to see your phone and visualize what it looks like and how it feels. OK, was everyone able to see all of it?

(Allow for responses.)

- Great! Now we are going to do some more visualizing, I am going to walk you through the same house, but this time, we are going to drop an item into each spot in the house that we stopped in. So, lets close our eyes and start at the door again, except this time, we are not just seeing the door, but we are seeing those carrots, which were the first item on the list. Visualize leaving the carrots on the floor by the door. Think about how silly those carrots look near the door. Take a good look at that door and those carrots. Now we are going back into the kitchen and we stop in the doorway again and look around. Right here, we drop the horse. Right in the doorway of the kitchen. Look at the horse, maybe imagine how big it is, how the kitchen is going to smell when you are done, how you are going to explain a horse in the kitchen. Take a second and look around. Now we visualize walking toward the refrigerator and standing in front it. Again, we are looking at the color of it, at the doors of the refrigerator, whatever we can see. I want you to see everything that you possibly can about the refrigerator. We drop the dog by the refrigerator. Maybe you can visualize the dog standing by the fridge and begging for some treats, but you walk away and leave him there and walk back toward the sink. You look at the sink carefully and, in the sink, you drop the cat. Maybe you can visualize how upset the cat is to be in the sink. Maybe you can feel the way the cat's fur feels as you pick it up and drop it in there. Again, you leave the sink because you realize you are thirsty and walk toward the cabinets where the cups are. You open the cabinet and what do you see? A cow! Maybe it is just the face of a cow in the cabinet and it moos at you as the door opens. Or maybe it is a tiny little cow. Whatever you see, you push it aside and grab a glass anyway and head back to the sink with your cup. Remember what's in the sink?

(Allow for responses; they should say that the cat is in the sink.)

- You push that silly cat aside and start to fill your cup with water, but instead of just the water shooting out of the tap, there are pickles coming out of it as well! Since you like pickles anyway, you shrug your shoulders, fill the cup with water and pickles and walk toward your bedroom and when you get there, you see that someone has filled the room with pencils. You figure it is someone trying to tell you to do your homework. You go to your computer or TV and see that you have left your phone on top of it and you wonder how it got there, but then remember that you put it there as something to remember for this list. You take your phone and decide that you are going to look at Instagram, but it seems that someone has hacked your account and all you see are pictures of babies. Now I am going to ask you again, who can repeat the list of items we talked about in order?

(*Allow for responses. Walk the students through the rooms again and prompt responses if needed.*)

- Wow! Look at that! You all used a memory trick to remember that long list of things that you might not have been able to remember otherwise. You all did such a great job remembering! Sometimes we can remember things just because we remember them, but other times it helps to use our memory tricks like we did today. Now we are going to finish our lesson with just one question. What do you think you are going to remember about today's lesson?

(*Allow for responses.*)

SELF-MANAGEMENT

Kindergarten to Third Grade

Materials:

    Markers
    Whiteboard
    Handout 6.1 – Managing My Feelings

Say the following:

- Today we are going to talk about ways to manage ourselves and our feelings. I'm going to read you a very short story and then we are going to talk about it. One day, Isabel was reading quietly in the reading corner. While Isabel was reading, Tiffany came over and grabbed the book away from Isabel. Isabel was very upset and told Tiffany to return the book. Tiffany ran away from Isabel and Isabel started to chase her. When Tiffany saw the Isabel was chasing her, Tiffany stopped, turned around and pushed Isabel to the ground. Isabel and Tiffany's teacher, Mr. Brown, told Tiffany that she was going to have to sit in the time-out area because of what she did. Mr. Brown also told Isabel that although she did not push anyone, she chased Tiffany after Tiffany took her book and for that she would also have to sit in the time-out corner. Who can tell the class what happened in this story?

(*Allow for responses.*)

- What do we think about the choices that Isabel and Tiffany made?

  (*Allow for responses.*)

- Let's talk about those choices. Were some of those choices bad choices?

  (*Allow for responses.*)

- Were some of those choices good choices?

  (*Allow for responses.*)

- What do you think the difference is between a bad choice and a good choice?

  (*Allow for responses.*)

- One good way to tell the difference between the two choices is to think about what might happen if you make a bad choice or what might happen in you made a good choice. What bad choice did Tiffany make in this story?

  (*Allow for responses.*)

- Right, Tiffany took the book, ran away and pushed Isabel. How do you know that this was a bad choice?

  (*Allow for responses.*)

- Right! One good way to tell that Tiffany made some bad choices is to think about what happened after she made her bad choices. What happened to Tiffany after she made her bad choices?

  (*Allow for responses.*)

- Right, she got into trouble and had to sit in time-out. Did Tiffany's behavior make things better or worse?

  (*Allow for responses.*)

- Right, her behavior definitely made things worse. What about Isabel? Did she make some bad choices too?

  (*Allow for responses.*)

- Yes, she did as well. Even though she did not push Tiffany, she did chase her through the classroom to try to get her book back. What happened to Isabel?

  (*Allow for responses.*)

- Right, she also got into trouble. Did her behavior make things better or worse?

  (*Allow for responses.*)

- Right, her behavior definitely made things worse because she got into trouble because of it. How do you think Isabel felt when Tiffany took her book away from her?

(*Allow for responses.*)

- What do you think Tiffany was feeling when she pushed Isabel?

(*Allow for responses.*)

- Those are all good feeling words that everyone came up with. So we know that both girls were feeling some very strong feelings when they made their bad choices. What could Isabel have done with her strong feelings instead of chasing Tiffany?

(*Allow for responses.*)

- What other choices could she have made once she dealt with her strong feelings?

(*Allow for responses.*)

- What could Tiffany have done with her strong feelings?

(*Allow for responses.*)

- What other choices could Tiffany have made once she dealt with her strong feelings?

(*Allow for responses.*)

- What about you? Have you ever made a bad choice?

(*Allow for responses.*)

- Did those bad choices get followed by something unpleasant?

(*Allow for responses.*)

- Were you feeling some strong feelings when you made those bad choices?

(*Allow for responses.*)

- We can see that very strong feelings sometimes lead us to make some very bad choices. Maybe it would make sense to find ways to deal with those very strong feelings so that it would be a little easier not to make bad choices. Today we are going to learn a bunch of different ways to deal with feelings and to make good choices. I am going to give you an example of something that I do to deal with some very strong feelings. When I feel those feelings, instead of making a bad choice, I try to take a very deep breath in and then let it out and then I take another deep breath in and then let it out again. What kinds of things can you do to deal with those very strong feelings so that you may not make bad choices?

(Write the following on the board: Managing My Feelings. Allow for responses and write these responses on the board. Make sure that the students come up with at least five viable ways to manage their emotions. Ideas for this could be walking away, taking a deep breath, counting to ten, tapping their finger against something, squeezing a stress ball or anything that the students can come up with that might help them manage their emotions in a positive way.)

- These are all wonderful ways to deal with strong feelings. I am going to hand out a handout that I would like you to keep so you can refer back to it when you need to. The sheet has a lot of these ideas on it. Now that you have your sheet, I want you to draw or write your own ideas to add to what is already there.

  (Allow time for students to add to the list.)

- Now that you have finished writing some of your own ideas, let's do a little practice to see what these ideas might look like if we were to actually use them.

  (Ask for a volunteer or pick a student and ask them the following question.)

- OK, let's pretend that you are Isabel, and someone comes and takes your book from you. How are you feeling?

  (Allow for responses.)

- Which one of those choices from the Managing My Feelings chart or handout will you use to manage that strong feeling you have when someone came and took your book?

  (Allow for responses.)

- Great choice. Now, what good choice are you going to make instead of choosing to chase Tiffany?

  (Allow for responses.)

- Good choice! What did _____ (name of student) do with those strong feelings?

  (Allow for responses.)

- What did that allow _____ (name of student) to do?

  (Allow for responses.)

- Great! Let's try it with someone else.

  (Go through each of the choices on the Managing My Feelings handout until all of them have been acted out and displayed to the class.)

- That is wonderful! You all did a great job. What I want you to do now is to think about a time that you made a bad choice. I will give you a minute to think about it. Does everyone have one?

  (Allow a minute for the students to think.)

• Great! Now, I want you to think about what feeling you were feeling right *before* you made that bad choice. What are some of those feelings?

   (*Allow for responses.*)

• Wow, such strong feelings! OK now we are each going to choose one of the choices on the Managing My Feelings chart and imagine that we used that choice to help with managing our feelings. Raise your hand if you think you might have made a better choice with the choice from the Managing My Feelings chart.

   (*Allow for responses.*)

• Great! What choice did you make?

   (*Allow for responses and make sure that everyone has a chance to share.*)

• Now that you all made such good choices, I am going to hand out paper and crayons and we are going to draw ourselves using the choice from the Managing My Feelings chart.

   (*Allow for responses.*)

• Excellent job! Let's share what we drew.

   (*Allow for responses.*)

• Everyone did such a great job learning how to manage their feelings. Who can tell the class why we should manage our strong feelings?

   (*Allow for responses.*)

• Who can tell the class one way to manage our feelings?

   (*Allow for responses and ask the question again until all of the choices have been said aloud.*)

• You all did a great job!

Name_____   Date_____

Managing My Feelings

I can:

1. Walk away

2. Take a deep breath

3. Count to ten

4. Tap my finger

5. Squeeze a stress ball

My own choices...

Handout 6.1

SELF-MANAGEMENT

Fourth to Fifth Grade

Materials:

>   Markers
>   Whiteboard
>   Handout 6.2 – If I am Feeling...

Say the following:

*   Have you ever felt like your emotions were getting the best of you? Like they were in control of you instead of you being in control of them?

    (*Allow for responses.*)

*   How does it feel when that happens?

    (*Allow for responses.*)

*   Today we are going to talk about ways to manage ourselves and our feelings, and we are going to start with a short story about someone

who was having some trouble managing their feelings. Jason was a young man who seemed to have some difficulty in school. He watched while all of his classmates seemed to learn how to read and do math so quickly and easily, but for him things seemed to move slowly. In fact, to Jason, many times it felt as if he were not learning at all. One night, while studying for a test for the next day, Jason decided that he was going to study for as long as he could to try to pass the test. He worked late into the night, but no matter how much he studied he could not seem to get the information he needed to remember for the test. When he woke up in the morning, he told his mom that he had studied for hours but was still not able to learn what he needed to learn for the test. As his mom was about to console him, his older brother interrupted and said, "That's because you're stupid." Jason jumped up from his seat at the table and pushed his brother to the ground. Their mom screamed at them to stop but not before Jason had punched his brother several times. What do you think Jason was feeling while he was having trouble studying?

(*Allow for responses.*)

- What do you think Jason was feeling when his brother called him "stupid"?

(*Allow for responses.*)

- What choice did Jason make after his brother called him "stupid"?

(*Allow for responses.*)

- Was this a good choice or a bad choice?

(*Allow for responses.*)

- How do you know?

(*Allow for responses.*)

- Raise your hand if you think that those feelings that Jason was having while he was studying and after his brother called him "stupid" might have had anything to do with his choice to fight with his brother?

(*Allow for responses.*)

- Jason's very strong feelings about studying and being called a mean name had a direct relationship with his choice to engage in the negative behavior of hurting his brother. Even though his brother was not right in calling Jason a mean name, Jason still could have chosen to find another way to handle the situation. The problem is that in the heat of the moment, sometimes, your decisions to engage in negative behavior seem to happen in a split second. That's why managing the feelings behind the behaviors is important. If we can get a grip on those feelings and manage them, then we can have a clearer head when it comes to making decisions that sometime get us into trouble. Who can share a time when they might have made a negative decision?

(*Allow for responses.*)

- What happened right before you made that negative decision?

(*Allow for responses.*)

- What feelings were you having right before you made that negative decision?

(*Allow for responses.*)

- So we can see that those very strong feelings can cloud our judgment. The trick is to deal with those feelings right when they are happening. What could Jason have done when he first started feeling those strong feelings while he was studying?

(*Allow for responses.*)

- Good. Maybe some other choices were to go talk to someone he trusts, or maybe walk away, breathe deeply, count to ten, listen to music or take a break. Recognizing that he is having those feelings helps him manage them and helps him make better decisions about his behavior. If Jason had been able to manage his feelings in a more positive way, what other choice could he have made when his brother called him that mean name?

(*Allow for responses.*)

- What about you? You all shared some experiences when you made some negative choices from some strong feelings. What could you have done when you started feeling those strong feelings?

(*Allow for responses.*)

- How might that have changed your choice to engage in negative behavior?

(*Allow for responses.*)

- Let's make a list of all of the things we can do when we start to feel negative and strong feelings. The idea is that if we can make those negative and strong feelings a little quieter, or if we can even replace them with positive feelings, then we may decrease the likelihood of making poor behavioral choices. So, let me give you an example. When I start to feel a strong and negative emotion, the first thing I do is name that feeling. Maybe I am feeling angry about something. Or maybe I am feeling really, really sad about something. It doesn't matter what it is, I first have to name it and acknowledge that it exists before I can try to make myself feel better. Once I name it, I usually try to take a very deep breath in and then let it out and then I take another deep breath in and then let it out again. If I am still stuck in those feelings, I might call a friend or take a walk. That way, if someone triggers me later on, I know that I will not lash out because I have already dealt with my feelings. So let's make that list.

(*Write the following on the board: If I am feeling _____, then I can _____. Model an example first such as, if I am feeling angry, then I can take a walk until I calm down. Allow for responses from the students until it seems clear that they understand what is being asked of them. After everyone has had a turn, hand out Handout 6.2 – If I am Feeling...*)

• The handout you were just handed will help you figure out more ways to manage your emotions and your behavior. Remember that first you have to name your feeling before you can find a way to deal with it. Let's take a minute to work on these handouts.

(*Allow time for students to work on the handout. Make sure to walk around the class and help students as needed.*)

• Now that we have finished naming our emotions and finding ways to deal with them, let's share.

(*Have students share their responses.*)

• Everyone did such a great job learning how to manage their feelings. Who can tell the class why we should manage our strong feelings?

(*Allow for responses.*)

• Who can tell the class one way to help deal with our negative feelings?

(*Allow for responses.*)

• You all did a great job!

Name_____   Date_____

If I am Feeling...

If I am feeling_____then I can_____
If I am feeling_____then I can_____
If I am feeling_____then I can_____
If I am feeling_____then I can_____

Feelings words:

Sad
Angry
Mad
Upset
Frustrated

Ideas for dealing with feelings:

1. Walk away
2. Take a deep breath
3. Count to ten
4. Tap my finger
5. Squeeze a stress ball

Handout 6.2

SELF-UNDERSTANDING: SMELL THE PIZZA

Kindergarten to Third Grade

Materials:

Handout 7.1 – Smell the Pizza
Markers or crayons

Say the following:

* Today we're going to talk about knowing yourself well enough to know when you're feeling nervous or scared about something. What are some things that make you nervous or scared?

  (*Allow for responses.*)

* What happens to you when you start to feel nervous or scared?

  (*Allow for responses.*)

* Is there anything you do that makes you feel better when you feel nervous or scared?

(*Allow for responses.*)

- When you are super, super scared or nervous do you think that it's easy to make good decisions?

(*Allow for responses.*)

- Sometimes students get really scared or nervous about lots of different things. Sometimes students might get nervous or scared about school, or sometimes students might get nervous or scared about home, or sometimes students might get nervous or scared about riding on the bus. People get nervous or scared about different things and it can be hard to figure out what to do when you start feeling like that. Does anyone want to share a time when they felt nervous or scared in school?

(*Allow for responses.*)

- Today we are going to learn a technique for managing those big scary feelings. I'm going to teach you a very special way to breathe so that you can manage those big scary feelings of being nervous or scared. Everybody breathes. It is something that we do naturally, and we do it all the time. We may not even realize that we're doing it. The kind of breathing I'm talking about is a little bit different than the kind of breathing we do every day. By breathing deeply and slowly we can help ourselves to relax and by helping ourselves to relax we can calm down those big scary feelings of being nervous or scared. I am going to hand everybody a picture. As soon as you receive your picture, I want you to sit as comfortably as you can in your chairs, and I want you to leave the picture on top of your desk.

(*Hand out Handout 7.1 – Smell the Pizza.*)

- Everyone should now have a picture of a pizza right in front of them. The first thing we are going to do is decorate our pizzas! I am going to hand out crayons and markers and we are all going to make our pizzas look as great as we can make them look.

(*Allow time for coloring in the pizza.*)

- Does anyone in this group like pizza?

(*Allow for responses.*)

- Great! Me too! Do you know what I like to do when I first see my pizza? I like to take a giant sniff of it because it smells so delicious. Does anyone else like to do that?

(*Allow for responses.*)

- Can anyone show me what that might look like?

(*Allow for responses.*)

- That is wonderful! I want everyone to take big sniff of their pretend pizza right now.

  (*Allow for responses.*)

- That was wonderful! How does everyone feel?

  (*Allow for responses.*)

- That is wonderful! The way we just breathed in that delicious pizza smell is the way that's going to help us when we get scared or nervous. I am going to teach you a special way to breathe by using the pizza and this kind of breathing will help you calm down when you start to feel scared or nervous. Are we ready?

  (*Allow for responses.*)

- OK, everyone make sure that your pizza is on the table. Lean over your pizza and close your eyes if you want to and hold a hand over your stomach. Take a deep sniff of the pizza – inhale through your nose with your mouth closed. You should feel your stomach rising like a balloon. Keep your shoulders from moving up too much. It should feel like you are breathing in that pizza smell deeply without moving too much of your body. Now let's count to three slowly in our heads while we are inhaling. When we reach three, open your mouth just a little and exhale slowly, also to the count of three.

  (*Demonstrate the breathing.*)

- OK, let's do it together. Ready? Smell the pizza.

  (*Demonstrate the inhale and count to three aloud.*)

- Now exhale through your mouth.

  (*Demonstrate the exhale and count to three aloud.*)

- How did that feel?

  (*Allow for responses.*)

- When we are in a stressful situation, remembering to smell the pizza can be a really helpful thing. Can you think of a time that smelling the pizza might have helped you to calm down?

  (*Allow for responses.*)

- Those are all good times to smell the pizza! Let's practice smelling the pizza one more time.

  (*Walk the students through another round of smelling the pizza.*)

- Excellent! Everyone did such a great job of smelling the pizza! Who can tell me what they will remember about what we learned today?

   (*Allow for responses.*)

- Great job everyone and remember to smell the pizza when you get nervous or upset!

Name_____   Date_____

Smell the Pizza!

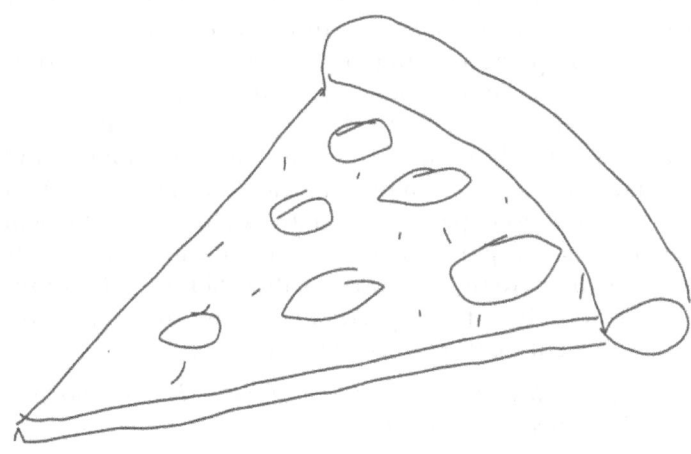

Handout 7.1

SELF-UNDERSTANDING: MY IEP

Fourth to Fifth Grade

Materials:

> Handout 7.2 – My IEP
> Copies of each student's IEP

Say the following:

- In this group, every single one of you has what we call an IEP. The letters IEP stand for the words individualized education plan. Everyone's IEP is different. That is why it is called an "individualized" education plan. Your individualized education plan is like a map to help you reach your goals. Each year your parents, teachers and your case manager meet to talk about how many of your goals you have reached. Some of you may attend your IEP meetings and some of you may not. At some point when you are older you will be required to be there. It is important to understand all of the things that are in your IEP so that you can become a better learner. One of the most important things to understand is what your learning disability actually is. Today, we will be discussing your IEP and what it means to you. Remember that everything in this group must stay confidential. An IEP is a confidential document and we must all make sure that we maintain that confidentiality. All IEPs have at least these four parts. They have a part called Present Level of Performance, a part called Accommodations and Modifications, a part called Goals and a part called Services. It is important to understand all of these parts. Let's open to the part of your IEP called Present Level of Performance.

   (*Allow for students to find the Present Level of Performance section of their IEPs. Help students as needed.*)

- What do you think this part includes?

   (*Allow for responses.*)

- This part lists your strengths and challenges and may also include test scores; observations; and comments from your teachers, parents or guardians and whoever else is involved in your education. Who wants to share some of your strengths as they are listed in your IEP?

   (*Allow for responses.*)

- Awesome! How about some challenges that you might have?

   (*Allow for responses.*)

- Great! It is important to know both your strengths and your challenges so that you can figure out what you need. Now let's look at the Accommodations and Modifications section.

  (*Allow time for students to find the Accommodations and Modifications section.*)

- What do you think might be in the Accommodations and Modifications section?

  (*Allow for responses.*)

- The Accommodations and Modifications section shows what accommodations or modifications the school has made to help you succeed in your education. For example, the accommodation section might have things like providing extra time for tests or allowing you to use speech-to-text software for writing. The modifications might actually change the environment, instruction or services so that your disability does not affect your learning. These things actually change the curriculum so you might be in special classes or may be learning things in a different way than students without IEPs. These accommodations and modifications are based on your own special needs. Does anyone want to share any accommodations or modifications that they are receiving?

  (*Allow for responses.*)

- Now let's look at the Goals section. What do you think might be in this section?

  (*Allow for responses.*)

- The goals section of your IEP is based on what you are going to need to accomplish. Why do you think it is important to know what is in the goals section of your IEP?

  (*Allow for responses.*)

- Right. The goals section of your IEP helps you monitor your own progress toward these goals as well. Does anyone want to share any of the goals outlined on their IEP?

  (*Allow for responses.*)

- Now let's look at the Services section of your IEP. Who can guess what might be in the Services section of your IEP?

  (*Allow for responses.*)

- The Services section of your IEP shows what services you are getting in your programming at school. For example, you might be getting speech services or occupational therapy services, or you might be going to a special classroom to teach you what you need to learn. These services will help you reach your goals. Who wants to share some of the services that you might be getting through your IEP?

(*Allow for responses.*)

- All of these things in your IEP work together to help you become the best you that you can be, but you need to have an understanding of what it is all about in order for this to work as well as it can. I am going to hand out Handout 7.2 – My IEP.

(*Hand out handout.*)

- This handout will help us to better understand what is in our IEP and how we can use this to become our best selves. Please start working on the handout as soon as you receive it and I will come around to help you as needed.

(*Students should be working on their handouts.*)

- Who wants to share their responses?

(*Allow for responses.*)

- Great job everyone! Who can tell the group why it is important to know what is in your IEP?

(*Allow for responses.*)

- Excellent! What is one thing you will remember from today's lesson?

(*Allow for responses.*)

- Wonderful! You have done a great job today learning about your IEPs!

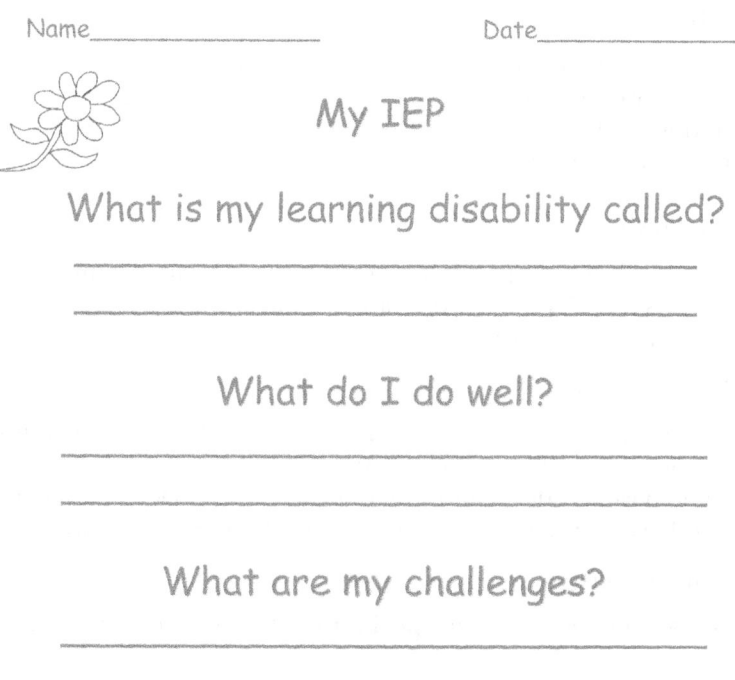

Name_____   Date_____

My IEP

What is my learning disability called?

_____

_____

What do I do well?

_____

_____

What are my challenges?

_____

_____

Handout 7.2

RESILIENCE

Kindergarten to Third Grade

Materials:

> Folder with a rectangle cut out in front to mimic a television screen, one for each student
> Handouts 8.1–8.7
> Crayons or markers

Say the following:

- Today we are going to talk about a very important subject. That subject is called resiliency or bouncing back. Has anyone in this room ever had a really hard day?

  (*Allow for responses.*)

- Everyone has a hard day every once in a while. The question is how do you bounce back? Some people are able to bounce back easily. Other people have a little bit more of a difficult time. Does anyone in this room have a difficult time bouncing back from a hard day?

  (*Allow for responses.*)

- Does anyone do anything special to help them recover from a bad day?

  (*Allow for responses.*)

- Sometimes when I have a bad day, I remind myself that bad things are temporary, and things will get good again soon. Sometimes when I need to remind myself that bad days don't last, I do deep breathing exercises like Smell the Pizza, the activity we did once before. Sometimes I try to act like a turtle. I try to pretend to go into my shell for a little bit and think about things until I feel better and then I come out. Today though, we're going to talk about changing the channel when you're having a hard time coming out of a bad day. I'm sure you have all changed the channel on your television sets before, haven't you?

  (*Allow for responses.*)

- Today we are going to learn how to change the channels on our emotions so that we don't get stuck in a bad place. I am going to hand out folders with the middle cut out, so it looks like a television set, and seven sheets of paper with different emotions written and drawn on them.

(*Hand out folders and worksheets 8.1–8.7.*)

- Each of the sheets has a different kind of feeling on it. The feelings are angry, scared, embarrassed, happy, neutral, sad and anxious. We are going to spend some time coloring our emotions the way we want them to look and decorating our television sets the way we want them to look as well.

(*Allow time for students to decorate sheets and folders.*)

- Great job everyone. Now I'm going to show you how this works. If I am feeling angry, then I put the angry sheet inside the folder, but I don't want to stay angry. I want to change the channel so that I feel better. I want to feel happy and because I can change the channel, I can take out the angry sheet and put in the happy sheet. I have changed the channel from angry to happy. This reminds me that I can do that with myself as well. Let's try it together.

(*Allow students to change emotions in the folder.*)

- I don't need to stay stuck in any emotion. I have the ability to get out of a negative emotion and jump into a positive one my television folder reminds me to do that. Let's think of a situation where you might be stuck in an emotion and you might need to change the channel.

(*Allow students to come up with situations where they may need to "change the channel."*)

- Great job everyone. Changing the channel on our emotions is a great way to be resilient and bounce back after we experience uncomfortable emotions. You don't need to stay in a bad place if you can change the channel! Let's wrap up now. What is one thing you will remember about today's lesson?

(*Allow for responses.*)

- Great answers! See you next time!

ANGRY

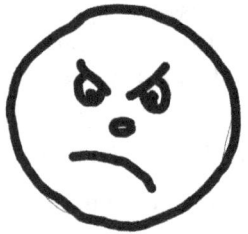

Worksheet 8.1

Scared

Worksheet 8.2

Embarrassed

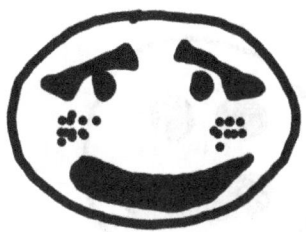

Worksheet 8.3

HAPPY

Worksheet 8.4

NEUTRAL

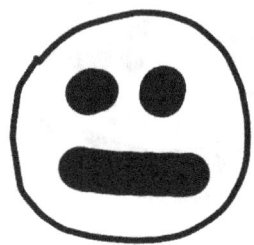

Worksheet 8.5

SAD

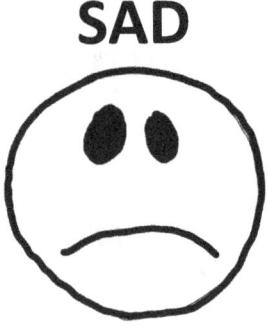

Worksheet 8.6

ANXIOUS

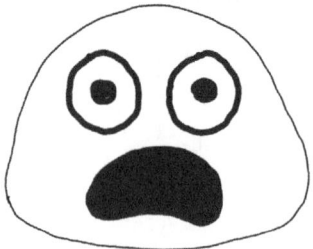

Worksheet 8.7

RESILIENCE

Fourth to Fifth Grade

Materials:

> Folder with a rectangle cut out in front to mimic a television screen, one for each student
> Handouts 8.1–8.7
> Crayons or markers
> Blank sheets of paper

Say the following:

- Today we are going to talk about a very important subject. That subject is called resiliency or bouncing back. Has anyone in this room ever had a really hard day?

(Allow for responses.)

- Everyone has a hard day every once in a while. The question is how do you bounce back? Some people are able to bounce back easily. Other people have a little bit more of a difficult time. Does anyone in this room have a difficult time bouncing back from a hard day?

(Allow for responses.)

- Does anyone do anything special to help them recover from a bad day?

(Allow for responses.)

- Sometimes when I have a bad day, I remind myself that bad things are temporary, and things will get good again soon. Sometimes when I need to remind myself that bad days don't last, I do deep breathing exercises. Sometimes I try to act like a turtle. I try to pretend to go into my shell for a little bit and think about things until I feel better and then I come out. Today though, we're going to talk about changing the channel when you're having a hard time coming out of a bad day. I'm sure you have all changed the channel on your television sets before, haven't you?

(Allow for responses.)

- Today we are going to learn how to change the channels on our emotions so that we don't get stuck in a bad place. I am going to hand out folders with the middle cut out so it looks like a television set, seven sheets of paper with different emotions written and drawn on them, and a few extra sheets for you to make your own if you need to.

(Hand out folders and worksheets 8.1–8.7.)

- Each of the sheets has a different kind of feeling on it. The feelings are angry, scared, embarrassed, happy, neutral, sad and anxious. We are going to spend some time coloring our emotions the way we want them to look and decorating our television sets the way we want them to look as well. We are also going to use the blank sheets to add any emotions that you might have experienced that are not covered in the worksheets.

  (*Allow time for students to decorate sheets and folders.*)

- Great job everyone. Did anyone have any other emotions that they used?

  (*Allow for responses.*)

- Great! Now I'm going to show you how this works. If I am feeling angry, then I put the angry sheet inside the folder. But I don't want to stay angry. I want to change the channel so that I feel better. I want to feel happy and because I can change the channel, I can take out the angry sheet and put in the happy sheet. I have changed the channel from angry to happy. This reminds me that I can do that with myself as well. Let's try it together.

  (*Allow students to change emotions in the folder.*)

- I don't need to stay stuck in any emotion. I have the ability to get out of a negative emotion and jump into a positive one. My television folder reminds me to do that. Let's think of a situation where you might be stuck in an emotion and you might need to change the channel.

  (*Allow students to come up with situations where they may need to "change the channel."*)

- Great job everyone. Changing the channel on our emotions is a great way to be resilient and bounce back after we experience uncomfortable emotions. You don't need to stay in a bad place if you can change the channel! Let's wrap up now. What is one thing you will remember about today's lesson?

  (*Allow for responses.*)

- Great answers! See you next time!

SELF-ADVOCACY

Kindergarten to Third Grade

Say the following:

- Today we are going to talk about self-advocacy. Self-advocacy is the ability to speak up for yourself when you need to. Self-advocacy involves making good decisions, knowing when you need help and being able to ask for it. It is important to know how to advocate for yourself in order for you to get what you need, but there are ways to stick up for yourself that might work and ways that might not work. Today we're going to talk about how to use self-advocacy in ways that actually get you the help that you may need. Let's start with a little story. One day, Jason's teacher, Mrs. Seltzer, gave the class some homework to do. Jason was really upset because school was sometimes hard for him and that particular bit of homework involved a lot of math problems that he did not feel comfortable doing on his own. Jason went up to his teacher and said, "You give too much homework! Why would you give us homework on stuff that you didn't even teach us? I'm not doing it!" What do you think about what Jason said to his teacher?

(Allow for responses.)

- Why do you think this?

(Allow for responses.)

- Jason is being very disrespectful to his teacher. What is he trying to tell her?

(Allow for responses.)

- Yes, he is trying to tell her that he is having trouble with the material, but he is not doing a very good job of it right now. How do you think Mrs. Seltzer felt when Jason spoke to her like that?

(Allow for responses.)

- Right! She might have been upset or angry.
- What do you think Mrs. Seltzer did after Jason spoke to her like that?

(Allow for responses.)

- So let's go back to what Jason was actually trying to say to Mrs. Seltzer. What was he trying to let her know?

(Allow for responses.)

- He was trying to let her know that he was struggling with the math and was scared that he would not be able to do it at home. So how could he have said it better so that he might have gotten the help that he needed?

(Allow for responses.)

- Those are all very good answers. Let's see what Jason did that actually helped him. One day, Jason's teacher, Mrs. Seltzer gave the class some homework to do. Jason was really upset because school was sometimes hard for him and that particular bit of homework involved a lot of math problems that he did not feel comfortable doing on his own. Jason went up to his teacher and said, "I don't think I understand the homework because I was having a hard time doing it in class. Can you help me?" What do you think Mrs. Seltzer might do now?

(Allow for responses.)

- Right! Mrs. Seltzer might give him help or maybe even give him different homework that he can do instead. How was Jason's second answer different than his first one?

(Allow for responses.)

- Yes, his second answer was respectful *and* asked for the help he needed. His first answer was disrespectful and blamed the teacher instead of asking for help for himself. Let's listen to one more story. One day, Sarah was sitting in class when her best friend, Cassy, took out a book and started to read it out loud. Sarah did not know how to read yet and started to feel embarrassed and upset that Cassy was able to. She started to cry and ran away from Cassy. Mr. Johnson, their teacher, saw that Sarah had run away from Cassy in tears and approached her. "Why do you look so upset, Sarah?" he asked. Sarah took a deep breath and said, "Cassy knows how to read and I don't and it made me feel really sad and embarrassed." What do think of how Cassy responded to Mr. Johnson?

(Allow for responses.)

- Right, Cassy responded respectfully and honestly. What do you think Mr. Johnson did next?

(Allow for responses.)

- Those are all great answers! Let's find out. Mr. Johnson looked at Sarah and said, "I know you feel bad, Cassy. It is hard when you see your friends learning things that you haven't learned yet. I can understand why it made you so upset, but just because you haven't learned how to read yet, doesn't mean that it is never going to happen. Some people bloom a little later than others. How about if instead of feeling bad about this thing you can't do yet, we go find something to do that you do really well right now? I've seen your drawings and I think you are a really great artist. Do you want to go draw some things instead?" How do you feel about how Mr. Johnson responded to Cassy?

(*Allow for responses.*)

- Right! Because Cassy was able to talk about her feelings and tell the truth about them, Mr. Johnson was able to help her figure out what she needed. Cassy did a great job of advocating for herself. Now let's do some practicing. I'm going to call each of you up to me one at a time. We are going to pretend that I am your teacher and that I am teaching you a new math problem that you are having a hard time understanding. I want you to pretend to be upset about it and maybe a little embarrassed or even angry, but I want you to tell me what you need in a respectful and nice way. I'll go first so that you can see what I mean. "Teacher, I am feeling really upset because I am having trouble understanding how to do these problems. I think I need more help with this. Can you help me?" OK, now it is your turn.

(*Call each student up individually and give them each a chance to ask for help in a respectful and kind manner.*)

- Everyone did such a wonderful job of self-advocating today! Who can tell us what it means to self-advocate?

(*Allow for responses.*)

- Great! Who can tell us why it is important to do it a respectful and nice manner?

(*Allow for responses.*)

- Wonderful! What is one thing you will remember from this lesson today?

(*Allow for responses.*)

- Great job everyone!

SELF-ADVOCACY

Fourth to Fifth Grade

Say the following:

- Today we will be talking about self-advocacy. Self-advocacy means that you are asking for the things that you need to be successful all on your own. So, as a very simple example, if you needed a pencil but you didn't have one, what might you do?

(*Allow for responses.*)

- Right, you would ask for a pencil. That one is simple. How did you know you needed a pencil?

  (*Allow for responses.*)

- Right, you did not have one. What would have happened if you didn't ask for the pencil?

  (*Allow for responses.*)

- Right, you might not have been able to finish your work. So asking for the pencil was a way of self-advocating. You knew what you needed, you asked for it and then you got it. But what if it wasn't that simple? What if what you needed was harder to figure out? In order to be a good self-advocate, you really have to understand what you are good at as well as what you may have challenges with. So let's start there. Who can tell me something that they are really good at? What is your biggest strength?

  (*Allow for responses.*)

- Who can tell me something that they struggle with?

  (*Allow for responses.*)

- Sometimes we don't want to admit what we struggle with because of lots of reasons. We might be angry that we struggle with it, or we might be sad, or we might even be embarrassed, but if we are not honest with ourselves and the people who can help us then we will never get the help we need to overcome our challenges. Great job talking about your challenges! I'm going to break you up into groups of two and give you a minute or so to tell each other your biggest strength and your biggest challenge.

  (*Break students into groups of two and have them tell each other their biggest strength and challenges.*)

- That was really wonderful. Let's go a little more in depth now and look at your academics specifically. Think hard before you answer these questions and be as honest as you can be. Here is the first question. Name three things that you do well in school.

  (*Call on one or two students and allow for responses.*)

- Name three things that you feel like you could be doing better in school.

  (*Call on one or two students and allow for responses.*)

- Name something that you like doing academically.

  (*Call on one or two students and allow for responses.*)

- Name something that you don't like doing academically.

  (*Call on one or two students and allow for responses.*)

- Great job! I want you to tun back to your partner and give you a minute to answer these questions with each other. I will write them on the board so that you can remember them.

  (*Give students some time to answer the questions with each other.*)

- Good job! Now let's look at how the answers to these questions work together when it comes to self-advocacy. I'm going to tell you a very short story and I want you to listen as I read it for the self-advocacy clues in the story. Vijay had a very good memory and could remember anything that was read to him really easily. One day, his teacher asked him to read out loud for the class, but Vijay had a problem. Even though he could memorize things, he really could not read well but because of his great memory, his teacher didn't know that Vijay was having trouble reading. Vijay could feel his face turning red and did not know what to do. Let's talk about this situation. What is a strength that Vijay has?

  (*Allow for responses.*)

- Right! He can memorize things. What is a challenge that he has?

  (*Allow for responses.*)

- Right, reading is a real challenge for him. What should he do next?

  (*Allow for responses.*)

- Let's read the rest of the story and find out what he does. Vijay was very upset and embarrassed and did not want the class to know that he could not read. He also did not want to get into trouble or to get his teacher mad at him. After thinking about it for a minute, Vijay told his teacher that he was having some trouble that he needed to talk to her about after class. What does Vijay need?

  (*Allow for responses.*)

- Vijay might need a few things. He might need more help with reading, and he might need his teacher to know that he is embarrassed by his difficulty with reading. How do you feel about how Vijay handled this?

  (*Allow for responses.*)

- Vijay was very respectful and was able to put himself in a position where he would not embarrass himself and would still get what he needed. Let's find out what happened next. Vijay's teacher could tell that there was something going on, so she did not push Vijay to read out loud right then. After class was over Vijay went to her and told her the truth about his challenges with reading and how he was embarrassed by it. Together they came up with a plan that would help Vijay get the extra help he needed to read. They also decided that Vijay would not be called on to read out loud in class unless he had his hand up and felt comfortable doing. How do you feel about how this was handled?

(*Allow for responses.*)

- What would you have done if you were in Vijay's situation? Why?

  (*Allow for responses.*)

- Have you ever been in a situation where you had to self-advocate?

  (*Allow for responses.*)

- Did you find it difficult to speak yourself? Why or why not?

  (*Allow for responses.*)

- Now we are going to work with our partners and create a story about someone who self-advocates. We are going to make sure that you answer the following questions that I will write on the board:
  1. What is your character's name?
  2. What is one thing that your character does well academically?
  3. What is one thing that your character does not do so well academically?
  4. What is a struggle that your character has?
  5. What does your character do to help themselves get over this struggle?

  (*Allow students time to come up with their story.*)

- Let's share our stories.

  (*Allow students to share their stories. Make sure that they return to the idea of self-advocacy as they discuss how their character was able to help themselves.*)

- Everyone did a great job creating and sharing their self-advocacy stories. Who can tell us what it means to self-advocate?

  (*Allow for responses.*)

- Great! Who can tell us why it is important to do it a respectful and nice manner?

  (*Allow for responses.*)

- Wonderful! What is one thing you will remember from this lesson today?

  (*Allow for responses.*)

- Great job everyone!

EMOTIONAL EXPRESSION

Kindergarten to Third Grade

Say the following:

- Everyone has feelings! Can you name some feelings that you may have had?

    (*Allow for responses.*)

- Great job! There are so many feelings! Let's see if you can guess what I am feeling right now.

    (*Do a charade of any easily acted out emotion, such as sadness, anger or happiness.*)

- Great job guessing!

    (*Do a few more to make sure that the children have an accurate understanding of what some of the basic emotions might look like.*)

- I think that you all did a great job guessing what I was feeling. Now it is your turn.

    (*Allow the students to each have a turn pantomiming some emotions of their choice.*)

- Great job everyone! Now we are going to talk a little more about those emotions you just named. It is important to be able to name your emotions so that you can make a decision about what you are going to do about them. For example, if I am feeling sad and I know that I am feeling sad, then I can say to myself, "I am feeling sad. I don't really want to be feeling sad right now. What are some things I can do to make myself feel a little better?" If I do that, then I can manage my emotions in a positive way. If I can't name my emotion, or if I don't really understand what I am feeling, what might happen?

    (*Allow for responses. Lead the children toward the idea that having emotions without being able to name or recognize them might keep you from being able to make yourself feel better. It might even get people mad at you if they don't understand why you are acting the way you are acting.*)

- It is important to be able to understand what you are feeling when you are feeling it. So let's talk about an emotion like anger. When I get angry, I feel like my heart starts to beat a little faster, like my thoughts are all happening faster than they usually do and like I am a balloon about to burst! Those things all let me name my feeling so that I can do something about it before I make a bad decision. What about you? What things happen to you that let you know that you are angry?

    (*Allow for responses.*)

- What about an emotion like happiness?

  (*Allow for responses. Keep asking the students the same type of question while substituting the emotions. Emotions you might want to include can be sadness, happiness, anger, jealousy, fear, guilt, grief, nervousness, annoyance and disappointment.*)

- Those are all great ways to know when you are feeling these emotions. Everyone did a great job. Before we end, who can tell me why it is important to be able to name your emotions?

  (*Allow for responses.*)

- Right! And for our final question, what is one thing you will remember about this lesson?

  (*Allow for responses.*)

- Great job everyone!

EMOTIONAL EXPRESSION

Fourth to Fifth Grade

Materials:

Handout 10.1 – Emotions Commotion!

Say the following:

- Emotions include things such as sadness, happiness, anger, jealousy, fear, guilt, grief, nervousness, annoyance and disappointment. Sometimes these emotions can get very complicated and sometimes you can be feeling more than one emotion at a time. When we feel these emotions, what we do about them has an influence on our behavior. So, for example, if I am feeling really sad and I am aware of the fact that I am feeling sad, I might express my sadness by crying. On the other hand, if I am feeling really sad but I don't let myself admit that I am sad, I might act angry toward people who are trying to be nice to me and that might lead to hurt feelings and maybe even a fight. It is important to learn how to identify and manage your emotions and learn how to express them appropriately. Let's start by trying to answer this question: What do you think I mean when I use the word "emotion" (or "feeling")?

  (*Allow for responses.*)

- Like we said before, emotions are things such as sadness, happiness, anger, jealousy, fear, guilt, grief, nervousness, annoyance and disappointment, just to name a few of them. These feelings can be caused by a situation or by people. For example, if I am with my friends and everyone is getting along and we are doing something fun, I would feel happy, but if I were with someone who was treating me badly, then I might feel angry or sad. What is one feeling that you have already had today?

  (*Allow for responses.*)

- If you feel comfortable sharing, can you share with the group why you might have had that emotion?

  (*Allow for responses.*)

- Great job everyone! Now we are going to talk a little more about emotions. It is important to be able to name your emptions so that you can make a decision about what you are going to do about them. For example, if I am feeling sad and I know that I am feeling sad, then I can say to myself, "I am feeling sad. I don't really want to be feeling sad right now. What are some things I can do to make myself feel a little better?" If I do that, then I can manage my emotions in a positive way. If I can't name my emotion, or if I don't really understand what I am feeling, what might happen?

  (*Allow for responses. Lead the children toward the idea that having emotions without being able to name or recognize them might keep you from being able to make yourself feel better. It might even get people mad at you if they don't understand why you are acting the way you are acting.*)

- It is important to be able to understand what you are feeling when you are feeling it. So let's talk about an emotion like anger. When I get angry, I feel like my hear starts to beat a little faster, like my thoughts are all happening faster than they usually do and like I am a balloon about to burst! Those things all let me name my feeling so that I can do something about it before I make a bad decision. What about you? What things happen to you that let you know that you are angry?

  (*Allow for responses.*)

- What about an emotion like happiness?

  (*Allow for responses. Keep asking the students the same type of question while substituting the emotions. Emotions you might want to include can be sadness, happiness, anger, jealousy, fear, guilt, grief, nervousness, annoyance and disappointment.*)

- Those are all great ways to know when you are feeling these emotions. Let's put all of this knowledge to work for us! I am going to break you up into small groups and give you each group some questions to answer. I want you to take about five minutes to look through the questions and answer them together. You and your partner may have different answers and that is OK. Write down any and all answers that seem right.

  (*Break students into small groups and hand out Handout 10.1 – Emotions Commotion!*)

- Who wants to share their answers?

  (*Allow for responses.*)

- Great job everyone. Who wants to share their favorite emotion to feel?

  (*Allow for responses.*)

- When are some times you feel that emotion?

  (*Allow for responses.*)

- What is your least favorite emotion to feel?

  (*Allow for responses.*)

- When was a time you felt that emotion?

  (*Allow for responses.*)

- We learned so much about emotions and why it is important to be able to recognize them. Before we end, who can tell me why it is important to be able to name your emotions?

  (*Allow for responses.*)

- Right! And for our final question, what is one thing you will remember about this lesson?

  (*Allow for responses.*)

Name_____   Date_____

Emotions Commotion!

1. How do you feel when you do well on a test?
2. How do you know you are feeling this way?

1. How do you feel when you don't do well on a test?
2. How do you know you are feeling this way?

1. How do you feel when you don't get invited to a party that all of your other friends have been invited to?
2. How do you know you are feeling this way?

1. How do you feel when you get to choose your favorite dinner to eat that night?
2. How do you know you are feeling this way?

1. How do you feel when you study really hard for a test but still don't do well?
2. How do you know you are feeling this way?

1. How do you feel when you don't understand something that is being taught in school?
2. How do you know you are feeling this way?

1. How do you feel when your best friend doesn't want to talk to you?
2. How do you know you are feeling this way?

1. How do you feel when you get in trouble for something you did not do?
2. How do you know you are feeling this way?

1. How do you feel when someone gives you a compliment?
2. How do you know you are feeling this way?

1. How do you feel when you are being hugged by someone who cares about you?
2. How do you know you are feeling this way?

Worksheet 10.1

SOCIAL SKILLS

Kindergarten to Fifth Grade

Materials:

> Index cards – Enough for each student to have a card for each member of the group. Each member should have as many index cards as there are members of the group. Each index card for each member of the group should also have that individual's name at the top.
> Pens, pencils or markers for writing or drawing

Say the following:

- Have you ever said anything mean to anyone?

  (*Allow for responses.*)

- Has anyone ever said anything mean to you?

  (*Allow for responses.*)

- How did it fell when someone said things that were not nice to you?

  (*Allow for responses.*)

- How do you think the person you said not nice things to felt when you said those things?

  (*Allow for responses.*)

- Today we are going to talk about how important it is to treat people with kindness and respect, and to be treated with kindness and respect by others. Let's go back to the questions I asked before about having been mean to anyone or having had someone be mean to you. Think about what your answers to those questions were and then raise your hand to answer this question: Who would you rather be friends with – someone who says nice things to you or someone who says mean things to you?

  (*Allow for responses.*)

- Someone who is nice to you can make you feel good and happy, right? So if you would rather be friends with someone who said nice things to you, how do you think other people feel about you as a friend if you say things that are not so nice? Today, we are going to practice saying nice things! I am going to start.

  (*Give a sincere compliment to each student in the group.*)

- How did it feel to get a compliment like that?

  (*Allow for responses.*)

- Is there anything about you that you would want someone to compliment? For example, I would want someone to compliment my intelligence! I would love for someone to tell me that I am really smart! What about you?

  (*Allow for responses.*)

- Today we are going to have an opportunity to practice saying nice things to each other. I am going to pass out index cards to each person. Each index card in front of you has your name at the top. Your job is to walk around the class and write or draw a compliment, or a nice thing about the person whose card you are writing on. Make sure that you go around the room to everyone and don't forget to give yourself one too!

  (*Hand out the group of index cards for each student. If there are ten members in the group, each member should have ten index cards. Each group of index cards should have that individual's name at the top.*)

- Does anyone want to share some of the compliments you got?

  (*Allow for responses.*)

- How did it feel to get so many great compliments?

  (*Allow for responses.*)

- Sometimes it is hard to remember how good it feels to have people say nice things to you, but making sure that we say nice things instead of mean things is really important. You might not want to be friend with someone who is mean to you and if you are being mean to someone, they might not want to be friends with you either. Saying nice things is important and makes people feel really happy! Who can tell the group why it is important to be nice and say nice things to other people?

  (*Allow for responses.*)

- Who can tell the group what they felt when they got those nice compliments?

  (*Allow for responses.*)

- What is one thing you will remember from today's activity?

  (*Allow for responses.*)

- Great job everyone!

References

Cortiella, C., & Horowitz, S. H. (2014). *The State of Learning Disabilities: Facts, Trends and Emerging Issues.* New York: National Center for Learning Disabilities.

Fitzpatrick, C., Archambault, I., Janosz, M., & Pagani, L. S. (2015). Early childhood working memory forecasts high school dropout risk. *Intelligence,* 53, 160–165. https://doi.org/10.1016/j.intell.2015.10.002

Rabiner, D. L., Godwin, J., & Dodge, K. A. (2016). Predicting academic achievement and attainment: The contribution of early academic skills, attention difficulties, and social competence. *School Psychology Review,* 45(2), 250–267.

Shapiro, D., Dundar, A., Huie, F., Wakhungu, P. K., Yuan, X., Nathan, A., & Bhimdiwali, A. (2017). *Completing college: A national view of student completion rates–Fall 2011 cohort.* Retrieved from National Student Clearinghouse Research Center website: https://nscresearchcenter.org/signaturereport14/

Index